MW01092099

Praise for *Weight Training Without Injury*

"Having studied the mechanics of injury for the past 20 years, I can attest to the importance of proper form with respect to resistance training. In this respect, Fred and Rachel have created a wonderful guide, appropriate for the beginner and professional alike. The authors provide a comprehensive, evidence-based manual that emphasizes correct form through user-friendly text and clear step-by-step instructions and photographs. The attention to detail is unparalleled among other texts in the field. If you were going to read and use only one book on weight training, this would be it!"
— **Christopher M. Powers, PT, PhD, FACSM, FAPTA**
Professor, USC Division of Biokinesiology & Physical Therapy

"It has taken me almost a lifetime to build a champion body. I have entered and won many competitions, most notably Mr. Universe. The key to achieve a champion body is to weight train consistently, with proper form to prevent injury. *Weight Training Without Injury* is brilliant—it educates the novice, as well as the professional, on how to train without injury."
— **Dave Draper, Mr. America,**
Mr. Universe, Mr. World in several competitions, 1965–1970
Author of *Brother Iron, Sister Steel: A Bodybuilder's Book*

"A clear and comprehensive guide, backed by scientific evidence and decades of real-life experience. A must-have for anyone needing to weight train safely—which is just about everyone."
— **Frank Winton, MD, Family & Sports Medicine**

"*Weight Training Without Injury* is an essential book for all ages to improve muscle strength and endurance without causing harm to the musculoskeletal system. The information presented is simple and concise, with formulas and schedules that are easy to follow. The chapter on proper squat exercise alone is so important that I have already changed the way I teach this exercise in my practice."
— **Stuart C. Marshall, MD**
Orthopaedic Surgeon, Specializing in Sports Medicine and Trauma

"*Weight Training Without Injury* is a tremendous resource for all types of athletes, fitness enthusiasts, and professionals. The methodologies in this book are sound, with scientific backing, and are presented in a very organized and easy-to-read manner. I definitely recommend this book to everyone that wants to train with great technique and excel in their respective fields."
— **Jon Sanderson, MS, CSCS, RSCC, SCCC, USAW, FMS, TPI**
Head Strength and Conditioning Coach, University of Michigan
Men's Basketball, Men's/Women's Golf

"*Weight Training Without Injury* is an indispensable, user-friendly guide, especially for the beginning lifter. The clear and simple instructions, along with the photos of correct (and incorrect) body positions throughout the range of motion for every step, make it possible to master proper technique when lifting weights—which is essential to avoid injury and maximize the benefits of resistance training."
        —N. Travis Triplett, PhD, CSCS,*D, FNSCA
        Professor of Exercise Science, Appalachian State University

"From beginner to professional, anyone can benefit tremendously from this book! Thanks to Fred Stellabotte, I not only know how to train effectively, but more importantly, how to train safely without injury. I have had the luxury of training with him, and if you wish to gain the same knowledge, this is the book for you. You will see the correct and incorrect way to train as if he were right there with you!"
        —**Richard Diaz, Arizona, USA**

"After months of physical therapy for my frozen shoulder, Rachel introduced me to the Complete Shoulder Move, featured in *Weight Training Without Injury* along with a wealth of invaluable training and advice. Rachel forever changed my life and healed my frozen shoulder."
        —**Eric Grotzinger, PhD**
        Associate Dean, Mellon College of Science, Carnegie Mellon University

"I absolutely love Stellabotte and Straub's book, *Weight Training Without Injury*! Having started fitness training in my early teens, in the weight room and in sports, I wish I'd had a guide like *Weight Training Without Injury*. Beginner, intermediate, and advanced lifters and trainers can benefit from this book as it demonstrates the right and the wrong way to do all the activities in the gym. It has a strong focus on feet and hand placement, head and neck alignment, spine and hip range of motion, and shoulder and knee joint stability. Science in the weight room—LOVE IT!"
        —**Stew Smith, CSCS, Former Navy SEAL, Tactical Fitness Author**
        Special Ops Team Coach at the US Naval Academy
        Founder of Heroes of Tomorrow and Stew Smith Fitness

"… Completely illustrated with high quality photos, this book leaves nothing to wonder about with regard to weight training…. This book [is] a bible for those involved in weight-training practice … [and] is an excellent companion for all athletes to achieve a thorough understanding of how to weight train—especially without injuries. The comprehensive notes accompanying each illustration and the index at the end elevate the status of this book to that of a reference manual, which is useful equally for the novice, professional, or trainer."
        —**Roy T. James for Readers' Favorite**

"Stellabotte, a personal trainer and veteran of the U.S. Navy, and Straub, an exercise physiologist, have built a clear and comprehensive manual that lays out the foundational basics of how to use weights and explicitly demonstrates the differences between safe, or 'correct,' movements and injury-causing 'incorrect' ones. The book is divided into seven sections, kicking off with a crucial introduction to selecting the right workout regimen. Subsequent sections focus on different parts of the body: legs, back, chest, shoulders, arms, and the all-important core. Along with the essential weight exercise for the body part in question, these sections go over necessary equipment, key points for safe and effective movement, and 'Master Techniques,' the more advanced exercises. The writing is clean and straightforward, effectively communicating what to avoid and what to do, as incorrect form can be dangerous. Color photographs appear on nearly every page illustrating the authors' tips. This guide is essential for anyone who hopes to get into weight training, and it should be mandatory reading before setting foot into any gym."
    —**Publishers Weekley**

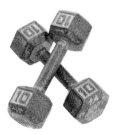

Weight Training Without Injury

Over 350 Step-by-Step Pictures Including What Not to Do!

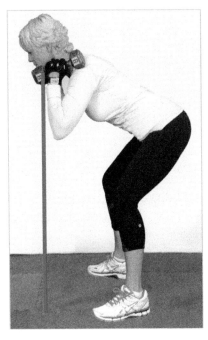 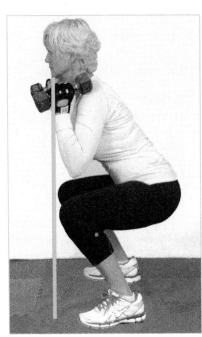

Incorrect   Correct

FRED STELLABOTTE • RACHEL STRAUB, MS, CSCS

REGALIS PUBLISHING

Important Notice to Reader:

The exercises in this book are intended for healthy individuals without any present medical conditions. If you are currently experiencing any bone, joint, or musculoskeletal pain, we advise you to consult a licensed health care professional prior to commencing a weight-training program. The authors, editor, and publisher specifically disclaim all responsibility and liability for any injury arising from the use and application of the information provided in this book.

Copyright © 2016 by Fred Stellabotte and Rachel Straub
All rights reserved. No part of this book may be reproduced or utilized in any form or by any means, electronic or mechanical, including photocopying or recording, or by any information storage and retrieval system, without written permission from the publisher.

ISBN: 978-0-9962638-1-8 (paperback)
ISBN: 978-0-9962638-4-9 (hardcover)
Also available in e-book format

Library of Congress Control Number: 2015937998

Published by Regalis Publishing, LLC
340 S Lemon Ave #6395, Walnut, CA 91789

10 9 8 7 6 5 4 3 2 1

Printed and bound in the USA

Editing and Book Design by Jill Ronsley, Sun Editing & Book Design, suneditwrite.com
Front Cover by David Savage Photography & Design, davidsavagephotography.com
Photography by Ahrend Studios, ahrendstudios.net
Exercises modelled by Vicki Stellabotte
Exercises photographed at the Stellabotte residence and Club Paradise Fitness, clubparadisefitness.com

Visit the authors at www.WeightTrainingWOI.com or contact them by sending an email to info@weighttrainingwoi.com.

 https://www.facebook.com/WeightTrainingWithoutInjury

 https://twitter.com/WtTrainWOInjury

 https://www.pinterest.com/WeightTrainWOI

 https://plus.google.com/+WeightTrainingWOI

 https://instagram.com/WeightTrainingWOI

To those who have needlessly injured
themselves while using weights and to those who
will be able to prevent injury through the use of this book
—Fred Stellabotte and Rachel Straub

CONTENTS

FOREWORD

THE NUMBER-ONE THING THAT YOU or anyone can do to improve your health is exercise.

Every January, millions of us make resolutions to join a gym, start walking, practice a sport, take up a martial art, or begin a training program. How many stick by these resolutions is the subject of many stories. Here is mine.

I have worked with Fred as my personal trainer for nearly 10 years. I had gone to him after a diagnosis of osteoporosis because I knew that I needed to perform weight-bearing exercises. And as a result of working out with Fred (combined with a course of medical treatment and clinical nutritionist-recommended supplements), my bone density did improve dramatically. Not only have I increased my overall strength, which is incredibly important as we age, but I have also improved my quality of life with regular workouts. Many of the exercises in this book are part of my regimen, and I have performed them for years and remained injury free.

I have also received so much more.

Fred's vast knowledge of the body and how to protect it from injury has led to an enhanced view of my best health practices. His expertise has been acquired from a lifetime of studying the human body. If I have any question about what to do for an ache or twinge here or there, Fred knows the move that will take care of it.

Within only six weeks of weight training, I knew Fred could also help my husband who had been recuperating from a second surgery on a herniated disc in his back. I knew he needed something more than the "don't lift anything over 10 pounds" that his neurosurgeon told him. I took him to meet Fred and I will never forget the relief I felt when he told me, "I can help your husband get strong enough that he should never have to have surgery on his back again." My husband has worked with Fred faithfully every week. He has performed the

1

majority of the exercises in this book and is able to continue his electrical business because he knows how to protect his back from further injury. Since working with Fred, he has taken trips into the mountains of Peru and hiked in the jungle. We are so grateful for his good health.

I met Rachel at the same time I started training with Fred, as she was there every day working with him as an intern. She was fascinated with his unique approach, which she wanted to document so others could benefit, too. The result of their collaboration is this wonderful book.

I have a profound appreciation for *Weight Training Without Injury*'s blend of Fred's immense experience with current supporting scientific evidence (there are over 90 references). Fred, a US Navy veteran, has been in superior physical condition throughout his life. His knowledge and experience result from years of research (including study with monks who practice martial arts in China; extensive coursework in kinesiology, anatomy, and neurology; and scrutiny of proper muscle function through examination of his own body in front of mirrors); personal application (which led to owning and operating the nation's largest gym facilities from 1970 to 1989, with over 13,000 members); and training others for over 50 years (the general public as well as professional athletes and bodybuilders, many of whom went on to win first place in major competitions, such as the San Diego Bodybuilding Open). Rachel's scientific research earned her three master's degrees: one in exercise physiology and another in nutritional sciences from San Diego State University, and a third in biokinesiology (with a focus on biomechanics) from the University of Southern California.

Fred and Rachel have achieved a truly remarkable training manual that provides step-by-step pictures for each exercise. But here's the most important part: additional pictures illustrate what *not* to do, which is a unique feature of the book.

This system is truly weight training without injury. Whether you are a professional athlete, a person like my husband who has had surgery and needs to know how to get stronger safely, or a person who just wants to become fitter, you will be able to reap great benefits from this book.

Linda E. Savage
PhD, licensed psychologist, and author of
Reclaiming Goddess Sexuality

INTRODUCTION

ORKING WITH WEIGHTS CAN BE ONE of the most beneficial things you do for your body. While the exercise itself will never hurt you, the way it is performed is crucial—improper form (using the wrong technique) will injure you. This is why correct weight training and information is essential, and that is exactly what this book provides.

Unfortunately, many people pick up weights with no idea of how to use them, and as a result, weight-training injuries are dramatically on the rise. Between 1990 and 2007, such injuries have increased by nearly 50% in the United States.[1] When we set out to write this book, we aimed to make it the most comprehensive book ever written on weight or resistance training for the public that teaches the correct method *and* shows the common injury-promoting pitfalls to avoid through the use of step-by-step pictures. And all our advice is backed up throughout by firm scientific research (over 90 peer-reviewed publications are referenced).

WHY WEIGHT TRAIN?

According to the American College of Sports Medicine, we should regularly engage in cardiovascular, flexibility, neuromuscular (balance and agility), and resistance training.[2] Of these areas, this book focuses on resistance or weight training—in particular, how to properly use weights and avoid injury. Weight-training benefits extend beyond improving physical strength and include reducing the risk of cardiovascular disease; improving body composition; increasing bone strength; reducing pain in those with musculoskeletal disorders; and improving mental health, fatigue, and well-being.[2]

We should point out that in this book "weight training" refers to the method of exercise that uses a range of resistances (for example, body weight, weight machines, and free weights) to increase muscle strength and endurance. We are not talking about the sport of weight lifting or competitive bodybuilding, both of which require training with generally heavy weights.

OUR MISSION

Our mission is to help you really understand the basics. That is why we begin each chapter with the Key Points for a Safe and Effective Exercise. Here we show the differences between injury-causing and safe movements using the terms "Incorrect" and "Correct." When neither movement is likely to cause injury, we use the terms "Correct" and "Correct (preferred)" to indicate the more beneficial method. We understand that everyone's lives are different, so we provide you with many options. Whether you wish to train at home with minimal equipment or at the gym with expensive machines, we show you how. However, with so many options, sometimes it is hard to figure out exactly what to do. That's why each chapter contains the Master Technique, Fred's personal recommendation for the best results.

WHAT TO DO (AND WHAT NOT TO DO)

Weight Training Without Injury takes you through the fundamental moves of weight training with over 350 step-by-step photographs, which show the correct methods *and* the common injury-promoting pitfalls to avoid. We show you what works, and what doesn't, and explain why.

This book is based on the training methods developed by Fred over the past 50 years and is complemented by extensive scientific research, so whether you are just beginning or are well established you can easily learn proper form and prevent injury.

UNIQUE EXPERTISE

Regardless of your training experience, we believe you will find the information in *Weight Training Without Injury* invaluable. The unique combination of expertise, clear explanations, and photos detailing what not to do for each exercise will, we hope, eliminate risk of injury and maximize the benefits of weight training.

Wishing you a safe and effective workout!

Fred Stellabotte
Rachel Straub, MS, CSCS
www.WeightTrainingWOI.com

Making Your Workout Efficient

*Working with weights can be the most beneficial
or the most detrimental thing you can do for your body.
The exercise will never hurt you—it is improper form that will injure you.*

How many days a week should I train with weights?

All healthy adults should weight train at least 2 days a week.[1] The American College of Sports Medicine recommends 2–3 days a week for novice training, 3–4 days for intermediate training, and 4–5 days for advanced training.[2]

How long should my weight-training session last?

We advise a minimum of 30 minutes. To obtain the greatest benefit, minimize the rest between exercises, which is called circuit training. This produces the greatest cardiovascular benefits.[3] If you can carry on a conversation, you are not working hard enough!

How should I structure my weight-training program?

You should regularly work each of your major muscle groups (legs, back, chest, shoulders, biceps, triceps, and core). Focusing on one group (for example, the chest) while neglecting the opposing group (such as the back) can lead to muscle imbalances and injury. For help with scheduling, see Chapter 2.

How many sets of each exercise are necessary?

Current recommendations are 2–4 sets for each muscle group.[1] These sets can be the same exercise or a combination of different exercises targeting the same muscle group. When your strength and technique improves, you can naturally increase your sets for better results.

How many repetitions for each set are recommended?

We advise 8–12 repetitions.[1] You can use more repetitions to improve muscular endurance. However, this is less conducive to increasing your strength.

Are 8–12 repetitions also recommended for core training?

Core training is the one exception to the standard 8–12 repetition rule. Core endurance, rather than strength, is most important for maintaining low-back health.[4] Therefore, the goal of core training should be high repetitions with low weight. No added resistance is needed. Perform as many repetitions as possible while maintaining proper form.

How much weight should I use?

If the last 3 repetitions of any set are not challenging, the weight may be too light. In that case, add more weight to increase the difficulty.

Is warming up necessary?

Yes. Warming up is important to prevent injury. One set with little or no weight for the move you are about to complete is sufficient.

How should I breathe during my workout?

In any activity, exhale on the exertion or the challenging part of the move. If you leave your mouth open and do not hold your breath, this should occur naturally.

How long should I rest between weight-training days?

Most muscles require between 48 and 72 hours to recover. Therefore, do not work the same muscle 2 days in a row. If you train with weights on consecutive days, perform a split-body routine; for example, train your upper body on day 1 and your lower body on day 2.[1]

Can I work my core every day?

The core muscles should be trained primarily for endurance, rather than strength. Therefore, they will recover quicker and can generally be worked daily. However, if your core is exceedingly sore, it is a good idea to rest a day or two before training again.

I am sore. Should I still work out?

Muscle soreness generally peaks within 72 hours. By this time, the muscle has had sufficient time to recover, so yes, you should train. As you become more accustomed to training, muscle soreness will subside. Actually, exercise helps ease pain by increasing blood flow, which removes waste products and increases endorphins.[5,6]

2

SELECTING YOUR INDIVIDUAL WEIGHT-TRAINING PROGRAM

There is no activity or sport that is not enhanced by proper weight training.

WHETHER YOU CAN ONLY TRAIN ONCE a week or want to do advanced training 5 times a week, this chapter will help you develop a suitable weight-training schedule.

PROGRAM FOR 1 DAY A WEEK

Don't be discouraged if you can only train once a week—it's worth the effort! Work your entire body using the following program.

Day	Workout	Recommendation*
1	Total body	Select 1 or more exercises for each muscle group. A sample schedule is shown on page 13.

* You can change this selection at your discretion, but a 30-day window is advised.

PROGRAM FOR 2 DAYS A WEEK

Work your entire body twice a week or perform a split-body routine; for example, train your upper body on day 1 and your lower body on day 2.

Total-Body Option (Preferred)

We say this program is preferred because you work each part of your body twice a week.

Day	Workout	Recommendation*
1	Total body	Select 1 or more exercises for each muscle group. A sample schedule is shown on page 13.
2	Rest	
3	Repeat day 1	

* You can change this selection at your discretion, but a 30-day window is advised.

Split-Body Option

Day	Workout	Recommendation*
1	Upper body	Select 1 or more exercises for each muscle group. A sample schedule is shown on page 14.
2	Lower body	Select 3 or more exercises. A sample schedule is shown on page 15.

* You can change this selection at your discretion, but a 30-day window is advised.

PROGRAM FOR 3 DAYS A WEEK

Work your total body 3 times a week or do a split-body routine (for example, train your upper body on days 1 and 3, and train your lower body on day 2).

Total-Body Option (Preferred)

This program is preferred because it allows you to work each part of your body 3 times a week.

Day	Workout	Recommendation*
1	Total body	Select 1 or more exercises for each muscle group. A sample schedule is shown on page 13.
2	Rest	
3	Repeat day 1	
4	Rest	
5	Repeat day 1	

* You can change this selection at your discretion, but a 30-day window is advised.

Split-Body Option

Day	Workout	Recommendation*
1	Upper body	Select 1 or more exercises for each muscle group. A sample schedule is shown on page 14.
2	Lower body	Select 3 or more exercises. A sample schedule is shown on page 15.
3	Repeat day 1	

* You can change this selection at your discretion, but a 30-day window is advised. Focus on your upper body in week 1 (as shown in the chart above), and concentrate on your lower body in week 2 (by making days 1 and 3 for your lower body and day 2 for your upper body).

PROGRAM FOR 4 DAYS A WEEK

Perform a split-body routine (for example, train your upper body on days 1 and 3, and train your lower body on days 2 and 4).

Day	Workout	Recommendation*
1	Upper body	Select 1 or more exercises for each muscle group. A sample schedule is shown on page 14.
2	Lower body	Select 3 or more exercises. A sample schedule is shown on page 15.
3	Repeat day 1	
4	Repeat day 2	

* You can change this selection at your discretion, but a 30-day window is advised.

PROGRAM FOR 5 DAYS A WEEK

Perform a split-body routine (for example, train your upper body on days 1, 3, and 5, and train your lower body on days 2 and 4).

Day	Workout	Recommendation*
1	Upper body	Select 1 or more exercises for each muscle group. A sample schedule is shown on page 14.
2	Lower body	Select 3 or more exercises. A sample schedule is shown on page 15.
3	Repeat day 1	
4	Repeat day 2	
5	Repeat day 1	

* You can change this selection at your discretion, but a 30-day window is advised. Focus on your upper body in week 1 (as shown above), and concentrate on your lower body in week 2 (for example, train your lower body on days 1, 3 and 5, while days 2 and 4 are for your upper body).

Sample Total-Body Workout*			
Back	 Cable Reverse Fly	Triceps	 Rope Pushdown
Chest	 Flat Bench Chest Fly	Biceps	 Preacher Curl
Legs	 Smith Machine Squat	Shoulders	 Complete Shoulder Move
Core**	 Stability Ball Plank Curl		

* Recommendation: Select 1 or more exercises for each muscle group.

** Generally, the core can be trained daily (as we explain in Chapter 1).

Sample Upper-Body Workout*			
Back	Cable Reverse Fly	Triceps	Rope Pushdown
Chest	Flat Bench Chest Fly	Biceps	Preacher Curl
Core**	Stability Ball Plank Curl	Shoulders	Complete Shoulder Move

* Recommendation: Select 1 or more exercises for each muscle group.
** Generally, the core can be trained daily (see Chapter 1).

Sample Lower-Body Workout*			
Legs	Smith Machine Squat	Prone Leg Curl	Dumbbell Lunge
Core**	Stability Ball Plank Curl		

* Recommendation: Select 3 or more exercises for your lower body.
** Generally, the core can be trained daily (see Chapter 1).

Weight-Training Tip

The sample exercise workouts we show in this chapter aim to help you determine an appropriate weight-training program. If you are just beginning, we advise you to start simply. Avoid overwhelming yourself with too many variations, as doing so may cause injury. Once you become more advanced, you probably won't need the workout cards at all.

SECTION II

LEGS

THE SQUAT

*If you had to pick one and only one exercise
to do for the rest of your life, it should be the squat.*

THE SQUAT IS A FUNDAMENTAL MOVEMENT. Not only is it crucial for daily living (getting in and out of a chair, for example), but is also one of the best exercises, if not the best exercise, for increasing physical strength. The squat causes movement at multiple joints and consequently strengthens and shapes major muscle groups such as the quadriceps, hamstrings, gluteals, calves, abdominals, and spinal muscles.[1] However, given the multi-joint nature of the squat, you have to take care to avoid injury at numerous locations.

During squatting, the knee (specifically the tibiofemoral joint) has to support loads of 5–7 times your body weight (compared with 2–4 times your body weight during walking), so squats can quickly damage your knees when done incorrectly.[2] Additionally, improper movements at your lumbar spine during squatting (such as excessive forward torso lean) increase the risk of low-back injury.[1, 3, 4]

Nonetheless, the squat is a safe and effective move if performed properly and can increase lower-body strength and quality of life.[3] This chapter shows you how to squat safely when using: (1) the Smith machine (a piece of training equipment with an attached moveable bar); (2) free weights (barbells or dumbbells); and (3) stable objects (such as a wall or counter).

EQUIPMENT OPTIONS

Smith Machine	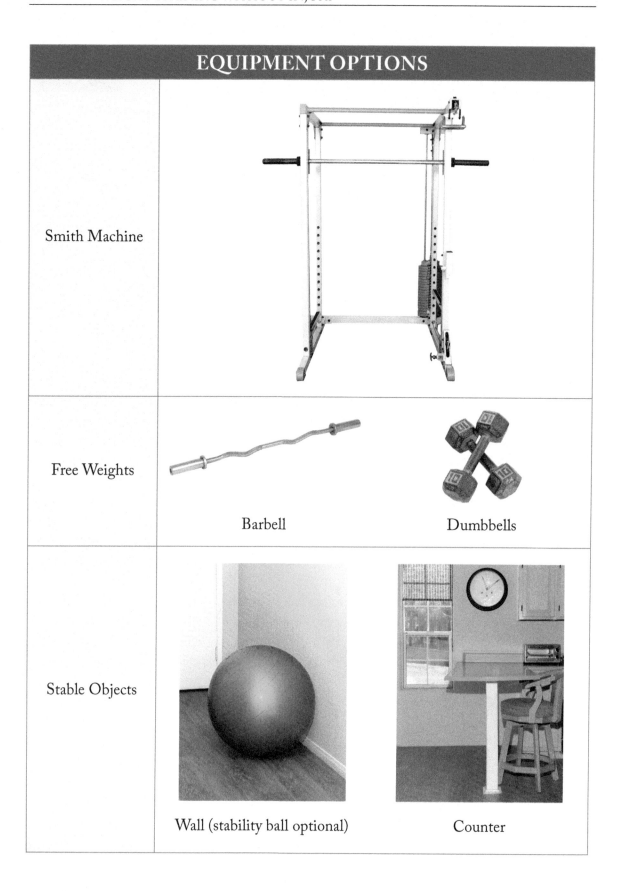
Free Weights	Barbell Dumbbells
Stable Objects	Wall (stability ball optional) Counter

KEY POINTS FOR A SAFE AND EFFECTIVE SQUAT

1. **Bar position (when using a barbell or Smith machine)**

   Place the bar on your back, *not* your neck. Please note: As we show here (and at various places throughout the book), gloves can be used. They are not a necessity, but they can help with your grip.

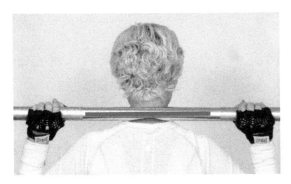
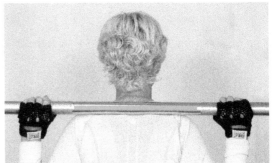

Incorrect	Correct

2. **Head position**

   Keep your head in an upright position with your eyes forward. Dropping your head promotes excessive forward torso lean, which increases the risk of low-back injury.[5] Extending your head back places unnecessary strain on your neck.

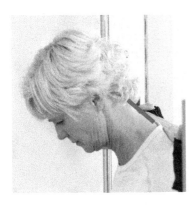
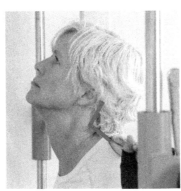
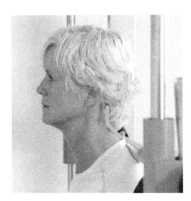

Incorrect	Incorrect	Correct

3. Foot position

Never place your feet straight. They should be rotated slightly outward. Rotating your feet outward increases your foundation and provides more stability. Use a shoulder-width or wider stance. Wider stance positions target your inner thighs and glutes (gluteal muscles, which make up your buttocks).[1]

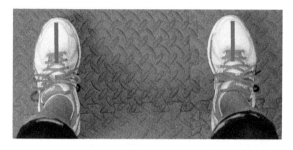 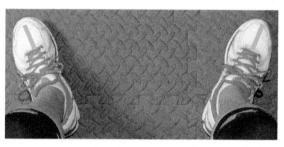

Incorrect   Correct

4. Knee position

Squat to 90° (or as close as possible). The top of your thighs should be parallel to the floor. Reaching 90° is the most effective method for targeting your quads (quadriceps, the muscles at the front of your thighs) and glutes. As you squat, activity in your quads and glutes increases.[3,6] If you experience knee pain, however, you may need to limit your range of motion so that pain does not occur—knee loading (particularly at the patellofemoral joint) increases as you squat.[7,8] If you can reach 90°, do *not* squat below this point. Going below 90° can damage your knees, specifically the articular cartilage and menisci.[1,9,10] Squatting below 90° does increase glute activity, but why run the risk of injury?[6]

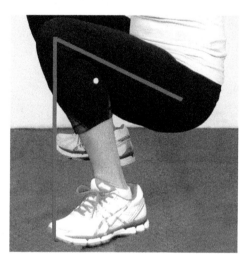 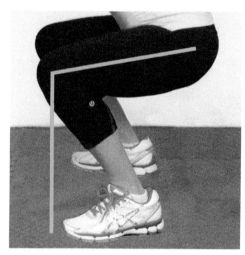

Incorrect   Correct

Avoid forward movement of your knees that exceeds the forward movement of your torso. Although it is generally advised that your knees not pass your toes to minimize knee joint loading (particularly to the anterior cruciate ligament and patellofemoral joint),[1, 11, 12] such a recommendation is incomplete as movement of your knees past your toes may be normal for you and no cause for worry.[13] To determine if the amount of forward knee movement is injury promoting, you must evaluate it in conjunction with the position of your torso.[14]

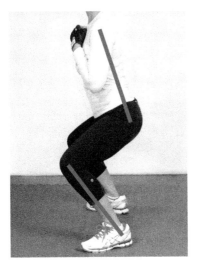 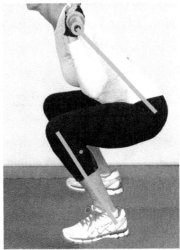

Incorrect   Correct

Keep your knees aligned with your feet. Letting your knees move inward places them in an unsafe position.

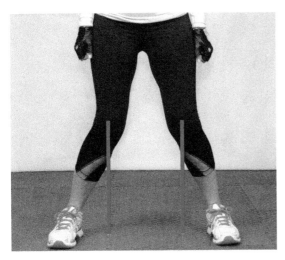 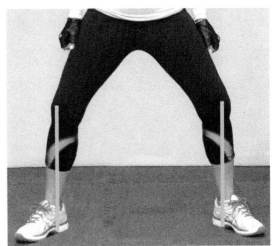

Incorrect   Correct

5. Back position

Keep your torso slightly forward to maximize glute activity and to decrease knee joint loading (particularly to the anterior cruciate ligament and patellofemoral joint).[3, 11, 12, 14] However, *avoid* allowing your chin to pass your toes excessively. Otherwise, low-back injury may occur from excessive forward flexion.[1, 3, 4] The spine, specifically the low-back (lumbar) region, is the most vulnerable joint during squatting, and as such, special care must be taken to avoid unnecessary spinal movements.[1] Nonetheless, depending on your anatomical structure (and the type of squat performed), slight forward movement of your chin past your toes may be unavoidable (particularly when using free weights, as shown in the "Correct" picture).

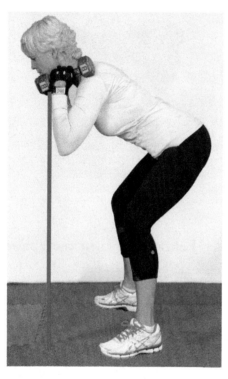
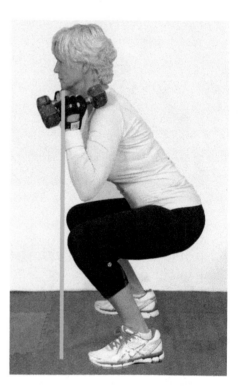

Incorrect   Correct

MASTER TECHNIQUE: SMITH MACHINE SQUAT

The Smith machine is the recommended equipment of choice for squatting. It provides stability, which reduces the risk of injury, and enables a complete (and more favorable) range of motion.

1. Start

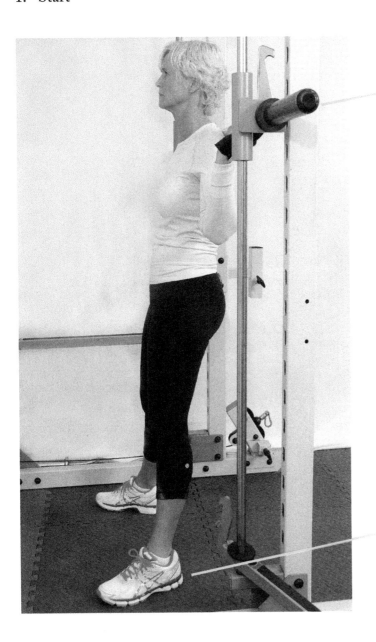

Bar position

Place the bar on your back, *not* your neck.

Foot position

Place your feet shoulder-width apart or wider in front of your body. Rotate your feet slightly outward.

2. Finish

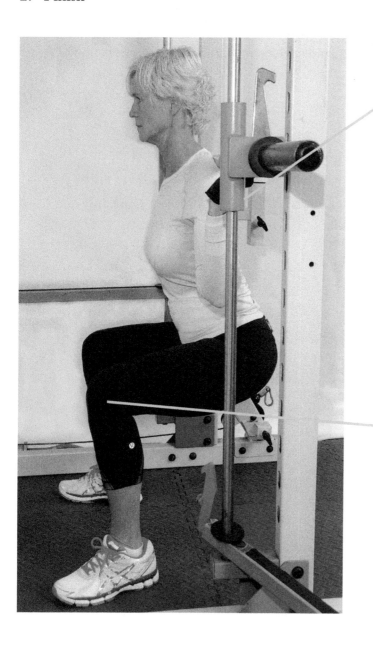

Back position

Keep your torso slightly forward. *Avoid* allowing your chin to pass your toes.

Knee position

Squat to 90° (or as close as possible) then return to the starting position. Keep your knees aligned with your feet. *Avoid* forward motion of your knees that exceeds the forward movement of your torso.

FREE WEIGHT SQUAT

The free weight squat produces greater muscle activity than the Smith machine version.[15] Be aware, however, that the instability provided by free weights increases the risk of injury.

Variation 1: Barbell Squat

1. Start

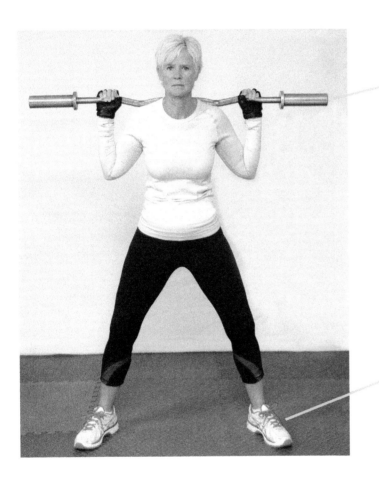

Bar position

Place the bar on your back, *not* your neck.

Foot position

Place your feet shoulder-width apart or wider. Rotate your feet slightly outward.

2. Finish

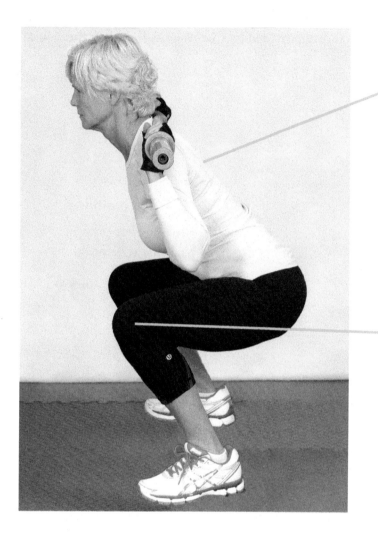

Back position

Keep your torso slightly forward. *Avoid* allowing your chin to pass your toes. However, slight forward movement may be unavoidable when using free weights (as shown).

Knee position

Squat to 90° (or as close as possible) then return to the starting position. Keep your knees aligned with your feet. *Avoid* forward motion of your knees that exceeds the forward movement of your torso.

Weight-Training Tip

For those with back troubles, avoiding free weight squats completely (such as the barbell and dumbbell versions) may be prudent, as they require the most forward torso movement.

Variation 2: Dumbbell Squat

1. Start

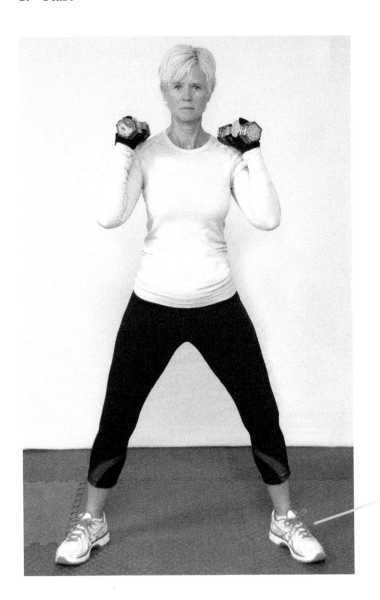

Foot position

Place your feet shoulder-width apart or wider. Rotate your feet slightly outward.

2. Finish

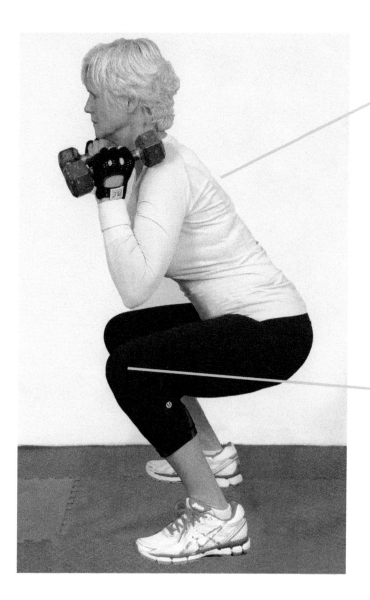

Back position

Keep your torso slightly forward. *Avoid* allowing your chin to pass your toes. However, slight forward movement may be unavoidable when using free weights (as shown).

Knee position

Squat to 90° (or as close as possible) then return to the starting position. Keep your knees aligned with your feet. *Avoid* forward motion of your knees that exceeds the forward movement of your torso.

SQUAT WITH STABLE OBJECT

The squat using a stable object is the least demanding.

Variation 1: Wall Squat

The wall squat can be accomplished with or without a ball. For added resistance, dumbbells can be used. Unfortunately, the wall lessens glute activity, as it restricts forward movement of your torso. However, placing your feet far enough in front of your body (such that minimal forward knee movement occurs) increases glute activity and lessens knee joint loading (notably patellofemoral joint compressive force and stress).[11, 14]

1. **Start**

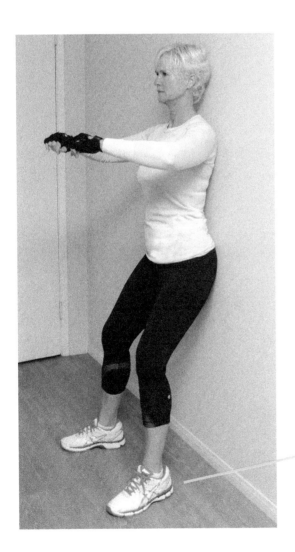

Foot position

Place your feet shoulder-width apart or wider in front of your body. Rotate your feet slightly outward.

2. Finish

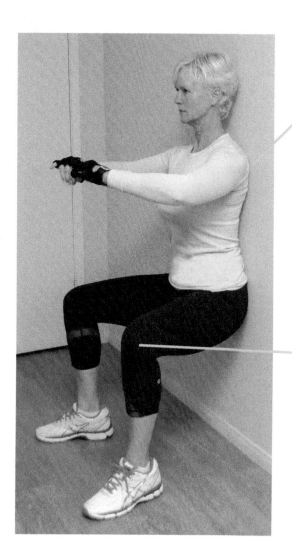

Back position

Keep an erect posture.

Knee position

Squat to 90° (or as close as possible) then return to the starting position. Keep your knees aligned with your feet. *Avoid* forward motion of your knees that exceeds the forward movement of your torso.

Variation 2: Counter Squat

The squat using a counter for support can be performed just about anywhere. Now you have no excuse for not squatting!

1. **Start**

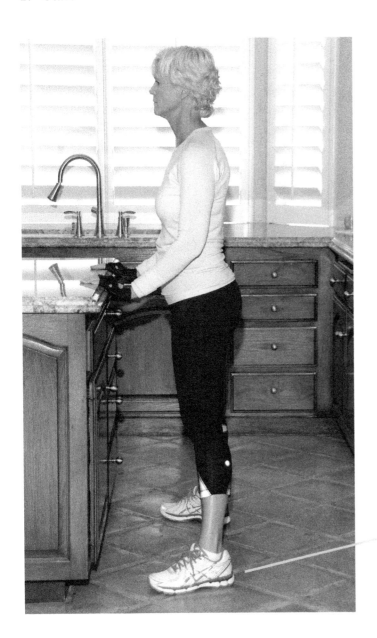

Foot position

Place your feet shoulder-width apart or wider. Rotate your feet slightly outward.

2. Finish

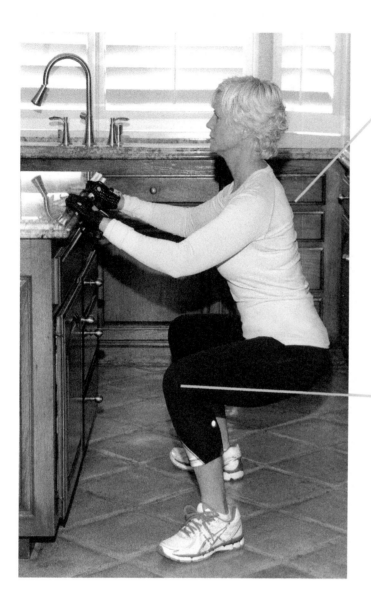

Back position

Keep your torso slightly forward. *Avoid* allowing your chin to pass your toes.

Knee position

Squat to 90° (or as close as possible) then return to the starting position. Keep your knees aligned with your feet. *Avoid* forward motion of your knees that exceeds the forward movement of your torso.

4

The Lunge

*The lunge offers similar benefits to the squat
but further challenges coordination and balance.*

THE LUNGE INVOLVES THE PLACEMENT OF one foot behind the other and can be performed stationary or while walking. Walking lunges, however, result in greater knee joint loading (specifically patellofemoral joint compressive force and stress).[1] Therefore, we recommend stationary lunges, which can be performed using either the Smith machine or dumbbells. Unlike with the squat, we do not advise using a barbell. It is too dangerous because it throws you off balance.

EQUIPMENT OPTIONS

Smith Machine	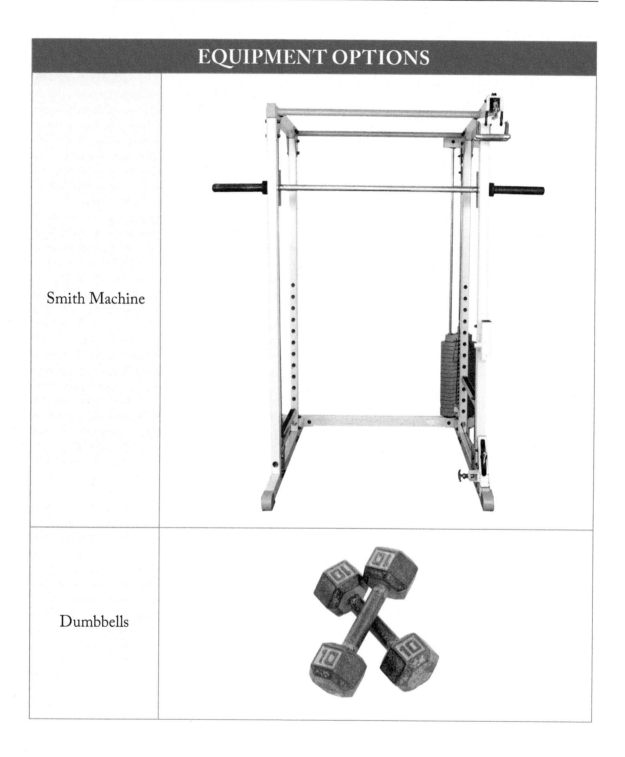
Dumbbells	

KEY POINTS FOR A SAFE AND EFFECTIVE LUNGE

1. **Bar position (when using a Smith machine)**
   Place the bar on your back, *not* your neck.

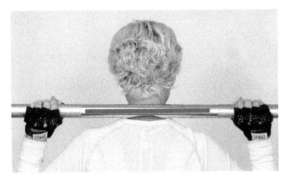 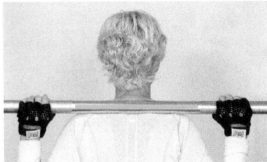

Incorrect   Correct

2. **Head position**
   Keep your head in an upright position with your eyes forward. As we discuss in "The Squat" (Chapter 3), dropping your head promotes excessive forward torso lean (increasing the risk of low-back injury), and extending your head back places unnecessary strain on your neck.

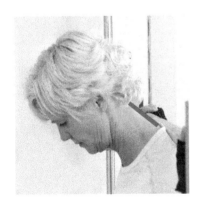 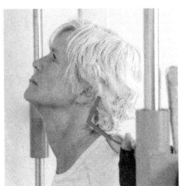 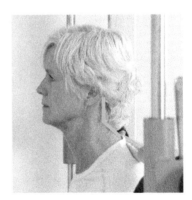

Incorrect   Incorrect   Correct

3. **Foot position**

   Keep your feet parallel during the lunge to maintain proper knee alignment.

Incorrect

Correct

4. **Knee position**

   Lunge to 90° (or as close as possible). As we explain in "The Squat" (Chapter 3), reaching 90° is the most effective method for targeting your quads and glutes. Remember, if you experience knee pain, you may need to limit your range of motion (in other words, go less deep).

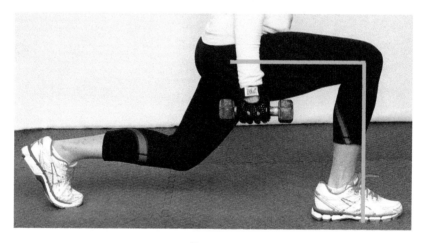

Correct

Avoid forward movement of your front knee that exceeds the forward movement of your torso. Allowing your knee to pass your toe increases knee joint loading (particularly to the anterior cruciate ligament and patellofemoral joint)[1-3] and is likely most problematic when forward knee movement exceeds forward torso movement.[4]

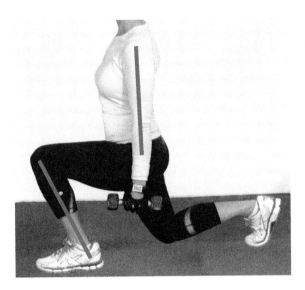 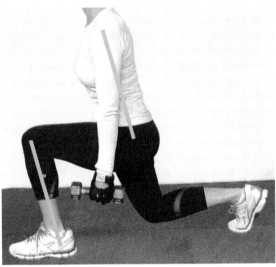

Incorrect   Correct

Keep your knees forward and aligned with your feet.

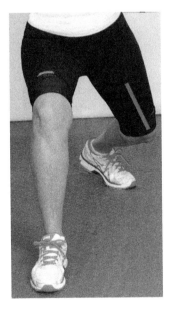 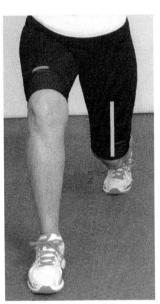

Incorrect   Correct

5. Back position

Keep an upright posture, but a slightly forward lean is normal. Low-back injury may occur from excessive forward flexion. Although lunging with a more forward torso increases glute activity and may decrease knee joint loading (particularly to the anterior cruciate ligament and patellofemoral joint),[3,5,6] such a configuration can be dangerous for your low back. Nevertheless, if lunging with a more forward torso is more comfortable for you, beware that if you experience any discomfort at your spine, you need to modify your posture to avoid injury. It is worth taking care because without proper technique the low back can easily sustain injury—the highest number of injuries among competitive lifters are in this area (23%), closely followed by the knees and shoulders.[7]

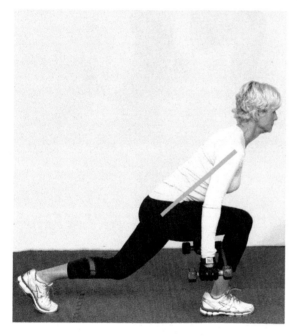 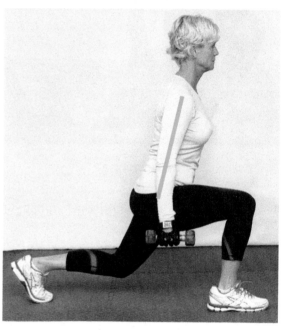

Correct   Correct (preferred)

MASTER TECHNIQUE: SMITH MACHINE LUNGE

The Smith machine is the recommended equipment of choice for lunging to ensure proper balance.

1. **Start**

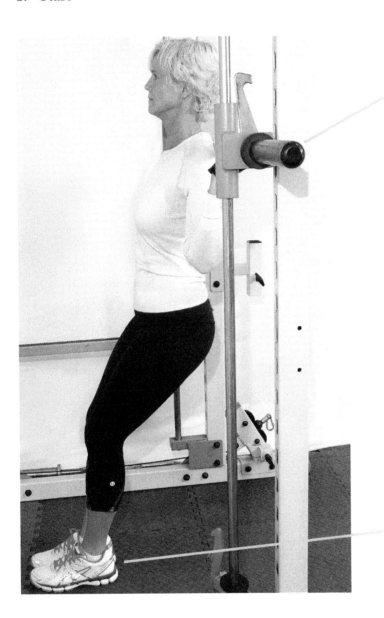

Bar position

Place the bar on your back, *not* your neck.

Foot position

Place your feet facing forward in front of your body.

2. Finish

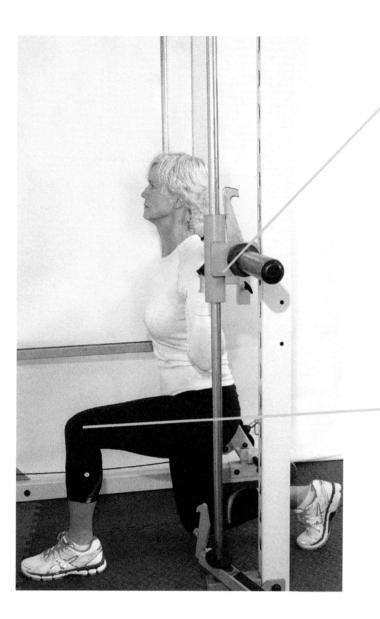

Back position

Keep good posture. A slightly forward lean is natural.

Knee position

Place one foot back and lunge to 90° (or as close as possible). Keep your knees forward and aligned with your feet. *Avoid* forward movement of your front knee that exceeds the forward movement of your torso.

DUMBBELL LUNGE

The dumbbell lunge should only be performed when you are stationary. Walking lunges are unsafe—you can not walk and place your feet perfectly every time—also, compared with stationary lunges, they produce greater knee joint loading (particularly patellofemoral joint compressive force and stress).[1]

1. **Start**

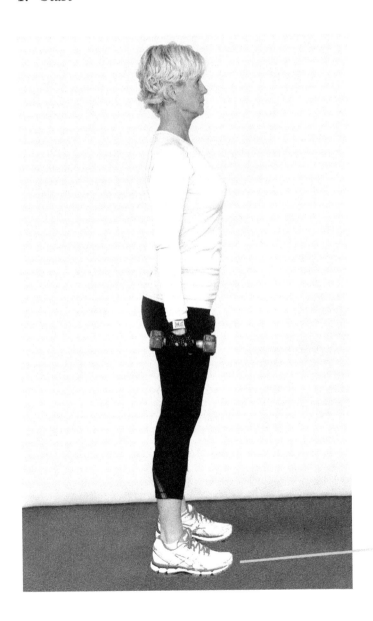

Foot position

Begin with your feet facing forward.

2. Finish

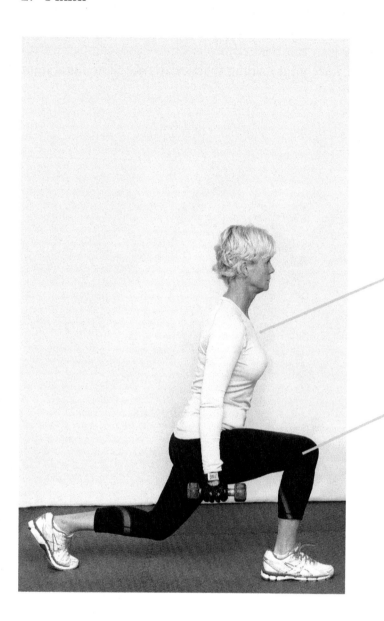

Back position

Keep good posture. A slightly forward lean is natural.

Knee position

Place one foot back and lunge to 90° (or as close as possible). Keep your knees forward and aligned with your feet. *Avoid* forward movement of your front knee that exceeds the forward movement of your torso.

THE LEG PRESS

*The leg press is easier to execute than the
squat, but injury may still occur from improper form.*

THE LEG PRESS, UNLIKE THE SQUAT, provides back support and places less force on your knees (specifically tibiofemoral and patellofemoral joint compressive forces).[1] Nevertheless, with improper performance serious injury can occur, particularly to your low back.[2]

In this chapter, when we talk about the leg press machine we mean one with a moveable foot platform and a fixed seat. There are two kinds, which we show you the proper use of: (1) the inverted leg press and (2) the seated leg press. These are the two types of leg press machines you will typically encounter. In this book, we do not cover machines with a moveable seat and fixed foot platform (often also called "leg press machines," confusingly), but the principles we outline in "The Squat" (Chapter 3) apply to this type of equipment.

EQUIPMENT OPTIONS

Inverted Leg Press Machine	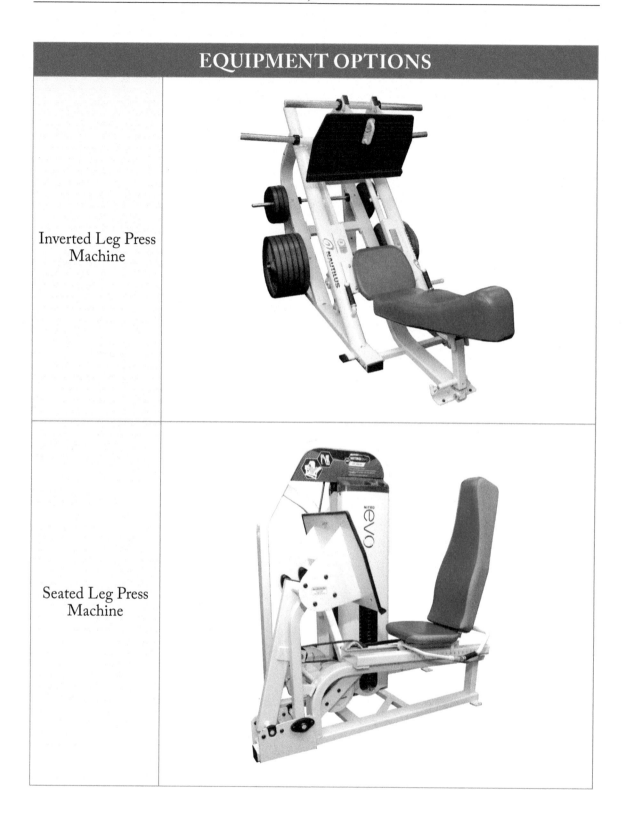
Seated Leg Press Machine	

KEY POINTS FOR A SAFE AND EFFECTIVE LEG PRESS

1. Seat position

Adjust the seat angle so your torso and thighs (when legs straight) create a 90° angle (or slightly less). This helps keep your low back in a safer position throughout the exercise. The inverted leg press (depending on the model) typically places you in the proper position.

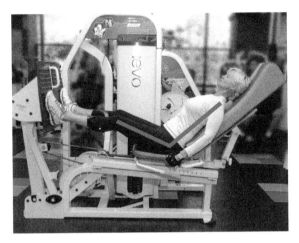 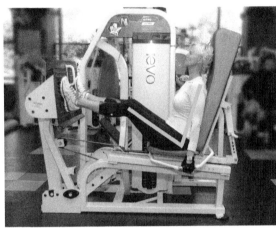

Incorrect	Correct

2. Foot position

Place your feet in the middle of the foot platform (or higher). Placing your feet too low may cause your knees to pass your toes during the exercise, which can increase knee joint loading. Also, higher foot positions target your glutes (while lower foot positions work your quads),[3] which helps unload your knees—improved glute strength protects against knee injuries.[4]

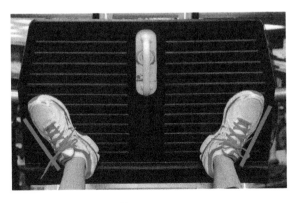 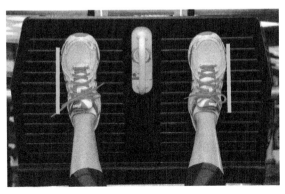

Incorrect	Correct

Preferably, use a shoulder width (or wider) stance with your feet rotated slightly outward. This allows for a deeper range of motion and emphasizes your glutes. And a wider stance allows you to bring your knees toward your underarms, protecting your ribs from injury. Bringing your knees deep into your chest can injure your ribs, particularly if using the inverted leg press.

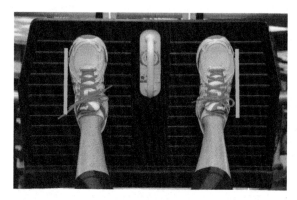
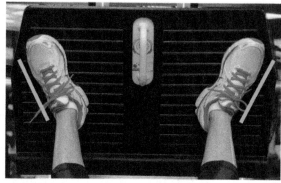

Correct   Correct (preferred)

3. **Knee position**

Bring your knees toward your underarms as far as possible. If using the seated leg press, you may need to slide the seat forward to obtain a fuller range of motion (though this depends on the model, as some models restrict the range of motion). However, we do not advise deeper movements if your low back rounds (see Back position, page 50).

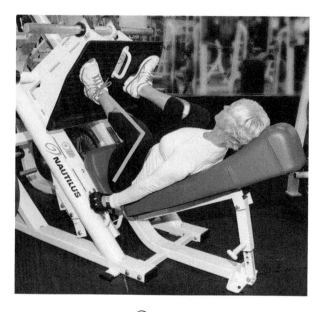

Correct

Keep your knees slightly bent. *Never* lock your knees.

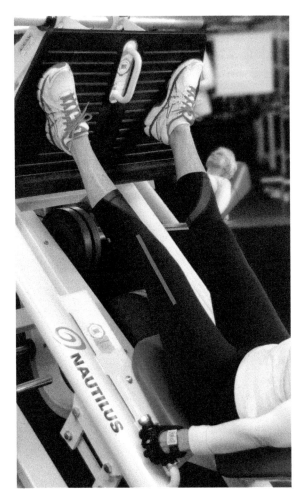

Incorrect

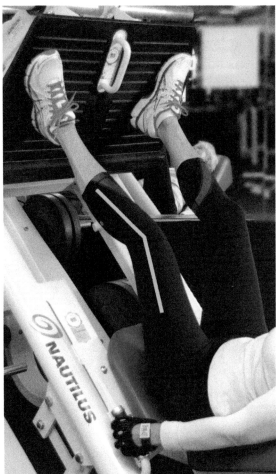

Correct

4. **Back position**

Keep your low back supported against the seat to maintain its natural curvature. Rounding your low back (to compensate for inadequate flexibility, core stability, or excessive weight) can lead to serious injury (such as disc herniation).[2] Generally, as you lower the weight, the likelihood of rounding your low back increases. Therefore, depending on your flexibility and core stability, you may need to limit your range of motion if you feel your low back rounding. This is difficult to show easily just with a photograph, so we are indicating the differences graphically between a rounded back ("Incorrect") and a well-supported back ("Correct").

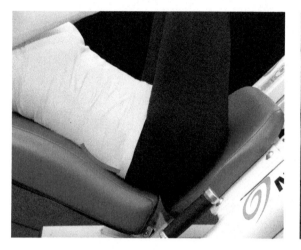
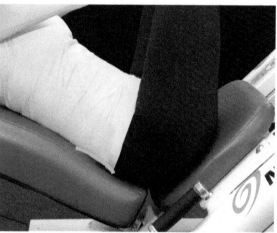

Incorrect   Correct

Weight-Training Tip

It is important to realize that you can injure your low back one of two ways: (1) excessive rounding (or flexion) or (2) excessive arching (or extension). For the purposes of this chapter, your low back is most susceptible to injury from too much rounding (as shown above). However, in other chapters (such as "The Plank"), it is most susceptible to injury from too much arching (as illustrated on page 241).

MASTER TECHNIQUE: INVERTED LEG PRESS

The inverted leg press is the preferred leg press machine. This machine provides a more stable back position and so allows a more complete (and safer) range of motion.

1. **Start**

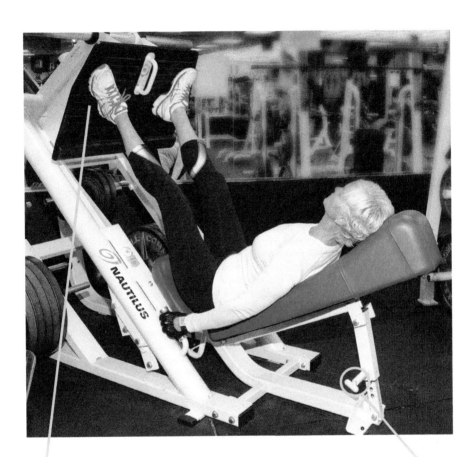

Foot position

Begin with your feet in the middle of the foot platform (or higher). Use a shoulder-width (or wider) stance with your feet rotated slightly outward.

Seat position

Adjust the seat so your torso and thighs form a 90° angle (or slightly less).

2. Finish

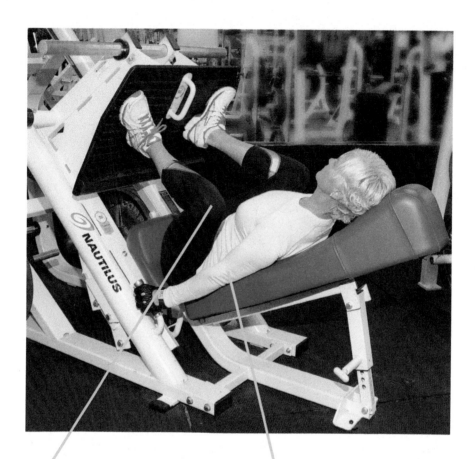

Knee position

Bring your knees toward your underarms. Then return to the starting position without locking your knees.

Back position

Keep your low back supported against the seat.

SEATED LEG PRESS

Compared with the inverted leg press, the seated leg press appears more attractive, as it places you in a more upright position. However, the more upright seat position tends to allow your low back to round more easily as you lower the weight.

1. **Start**

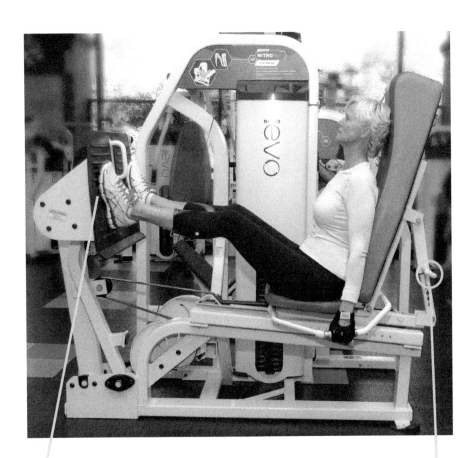

Foot position

Begin with your feet in the middle of the foot platform (or higher). Use a shoulder width (or wider) stance with your feet rotated slightly outward.

Seat position

Adjust the seat so your torso and thighs form a 90° angle (or slightly less).

2. Finish

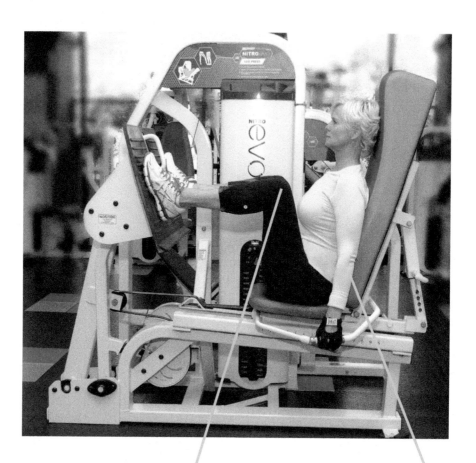

Knee position

Bring your knees toward your underarms. Then return to the starting position without locking your knees.

Back position

Keep your low back supported against the seat.

The Leg Extension

The leg extension allows you to strengthen your quads in a seated position. Stability is no longer an issue, and potential strain on your low back is eliminated.

THE LEG EXTENSION HAS ATTAINED A bad reputation among fitness professionals because it isolates your quads and potentially places dangerous loads on your knees. However, the leg extension's bad reputation is not warranted. Current research shows that individuals with knee pathologies benefit from squatting *and* knee extension exercises.[1,2]

Knee loading (specifically patellofemoral joint stress) is in fact *lower* with the leg extension from approximately 45° to 90°.[3,4] Therefore, if you can't reach a 90° knee angle with the squat to target your quads, you now have a second option—the leg extension!

EQUIPMENT OPTIONS

Leg Extension
Machine

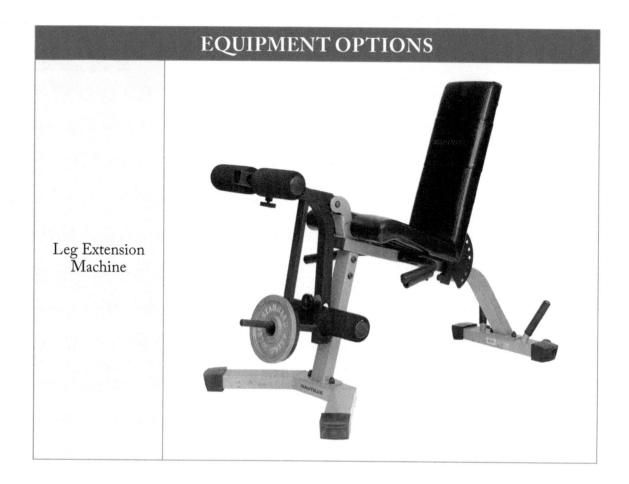

Weight-Training Tip

*If you do not have access to a leg extension machine,
you could use ankle weights. But a better use of your time would
be to forgo this exercise and instead perform a squat, lunge, or leg press.*

KEY POINTS FOR A SAFE
AND EFFECTIVE LEG EXTENSION

1. Knee position

Bend your knees to 90° (or as close as possible) but *never* more. Otherwise, you may injure your knees (the menisci, for example).[5-7]

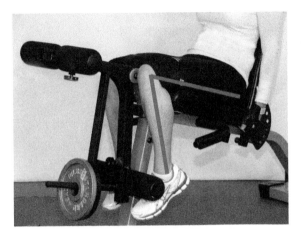

Incorrect

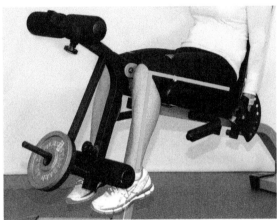

Correct

Do *not* lock your knees. Extending your legs to such a position results in the highest knee joint loading (notably patellofemoral joint stress).[4,8] However, if you experience knee pain, you may need to even further limit your range of motion. Knee loading increases as your legs straighten (whereas, in the squat, knee loading increases as your knees bend).[4]

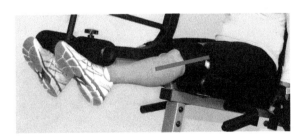

Incorrect

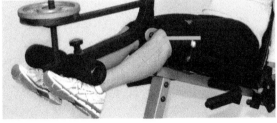

Correct

MASTER TECHNIQUE: SEATED LEG EXTENSION

1. **Start**

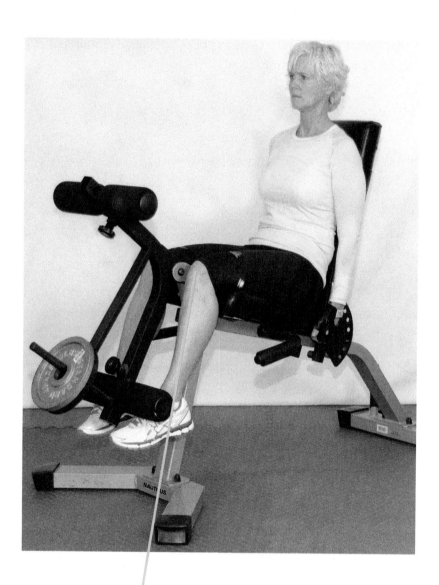

Knee position

Bend your knees to 90°
(or as close as possible)
but *never* more.

2. Finish

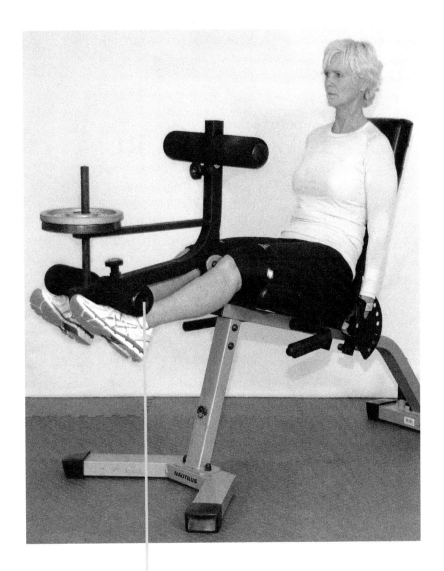

Weight position

Bring the weight upward without locking your knees.

7

THE LEG CURL

The hamstrings are not to be neglected.
Frequently people have strong quads (front thigh muscles), but weak
hamstrings (back thigh muscles), which predisposes the hamstrings to injury.

THE HAMSTRINGS ARE THE MAIN PLACE of injury in numerous sports; for example, they account for approximately 26% of all track and field injuries. While there are many causes of hamstring injuries, strength imbalances (specifically, having stronger quads than hamstrings) predispose the hamstrings to injury.[1]

Although the squat is consistently used to strengthen the leg musculature, research suggests that the exercise produces minimal hamstring activity.[2] So, in this chapter, we demonstrate proper hamstring strengthening—specifically with the leg curl.

EQUIPMENT OPTIONS

Prone Leg Curl Machine	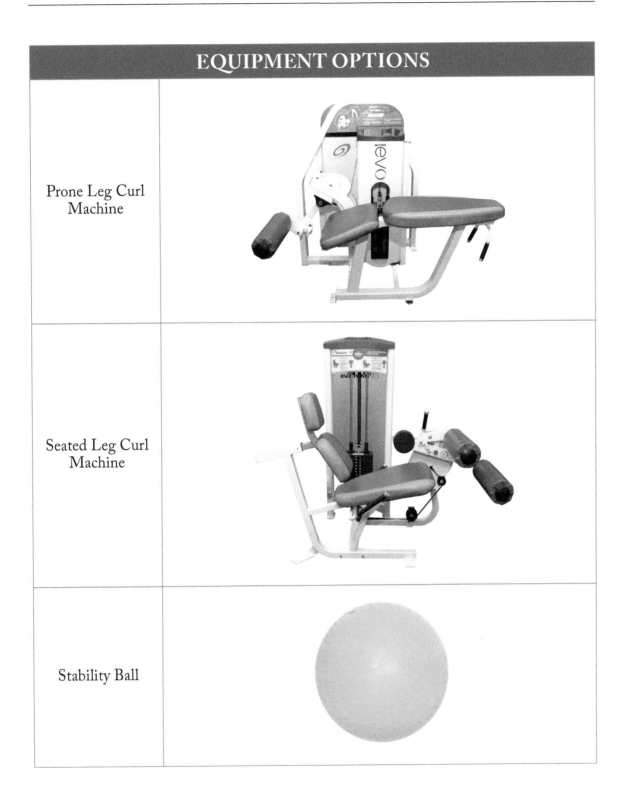
Seated Leg Curl Machine	
Stability Ball	

KEY POINTS FOR A SAFE AND EFFECTIVE LEG CURL

1. Exercises to be avoided

Avoid deadlifts (hamstring exercises, which require you to bend repetitively at the waist). Debilitating back injuries can result if your form isn't perfect, particularly if a heavy weight is used—leave it for the professionals![3] Please note: Although deadlifts are not technically leg curl exercises, we are telling you here to avoid deadlifts since this is the only chapter dedicated to hamstring strengthening.

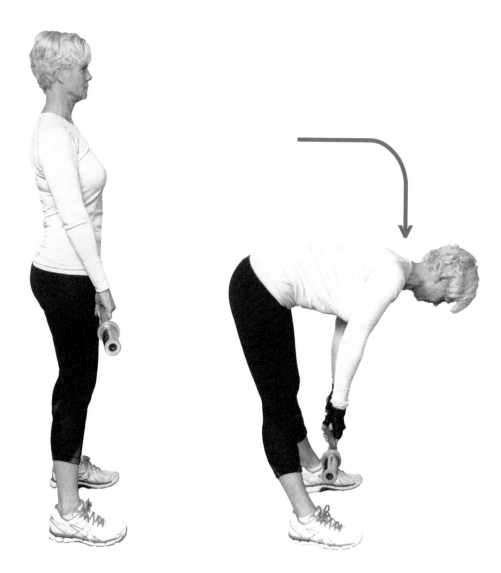

Deadlift (to be avoided)

2. **Head position (when using a prone leg curl machine)**

Keep your head in a natural position. If you're lying face down, place your head on its side to avoid neck strain.

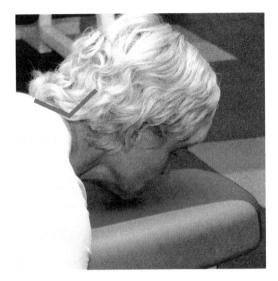
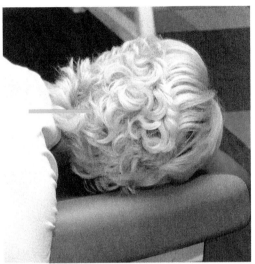

Incorrect   Correct

3. **Knee position**

Keep your knees slightly bent. *Never* lock your knees.

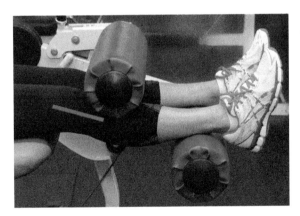
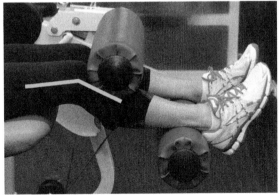

Incorrect   Correct

MASTER TECHNIQUE: PRONE LEG CURL

The prone leg curl is the preferred curl for hamstring strengthening. It enables a full range of motion and is easily adjusted for different body types. To get the maximum benefit from this move, lower the weight in a controlled manner after curling the weight. This is particularly important since most hamstring injuries occur from inadequate strength in the lowering (eccentric) phase.[4,5]

1. **Start**

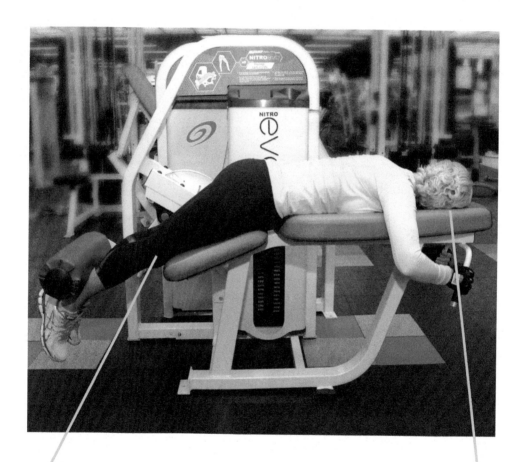

Knee position

Begin with your legs extended and your knees slightly bent.

Head position

Place your head on its side.

2. Finish

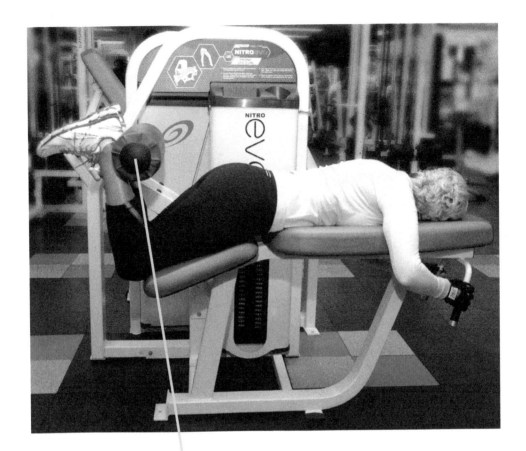

Weight position

Curl the weight toward your glutes as far as possible (without raising your glutes). Then slowly lower the weight to the starting position.

SEATED LEG CURL

The benefit of the seated leg curl is that it lessens strain on your low back. However, obtaining a full range of motion is not always possible—it depends on the machine's design. As you did for the prone leg curl, control the weight as your legs straighten.

1. Start

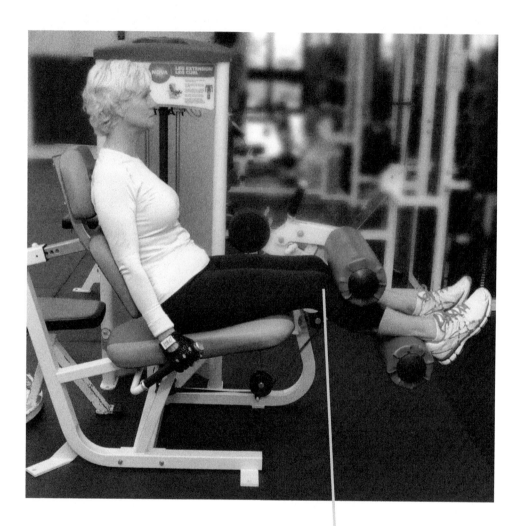

Knee position

Begin with your legs extended and your knees slightly bent.

2. Finish

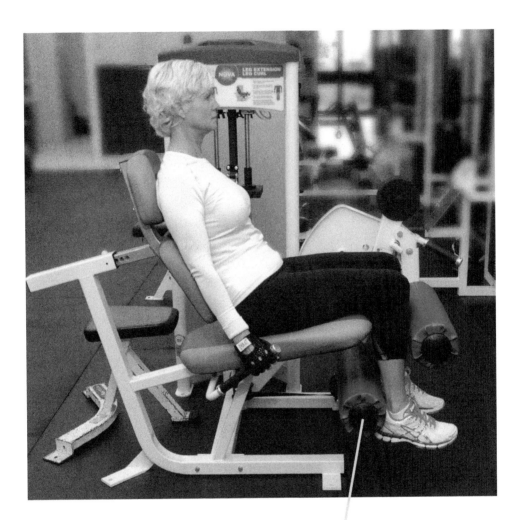

Weight position

Curl the weight toward your glutes as far as possible (while keeping your thighs firmly against the seat). Then slowly return the weight to the starting position.

STABILITY BALL LEG CURL

The stability ball leg curl requires no machine and has the added benefit of being a core exercise.

1. Start

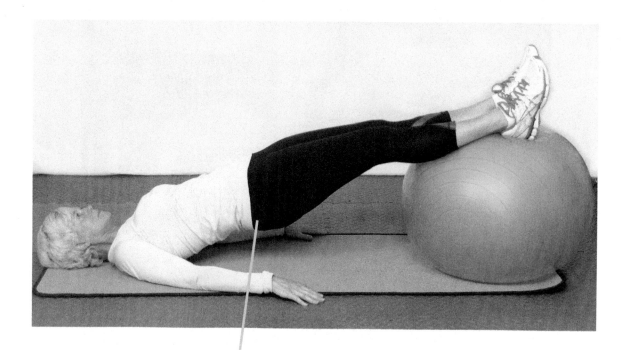

Hip position

Raise your hips. Practice this position until you're stable before curling the ball.

2. Finish

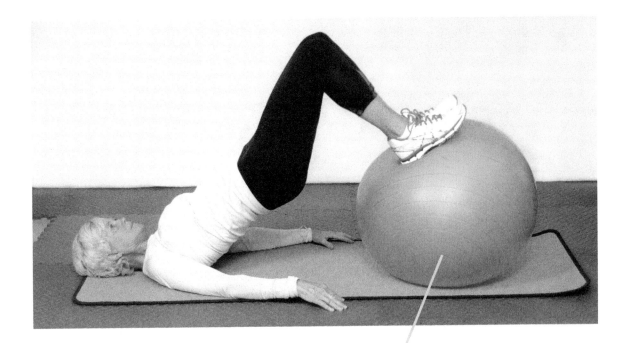

Ball position

Curl the ball toward your glutes as far as possible (while keeping your hips raised). Then slowly return the ball to the starting position.

THE CALF RAISE

---

*Any movement that raises the heel upward employs
the calf, yet the calf is one of the most difficult muscles to develop.*

THE MAIN PROBLEM THAT AFFECTS THE calf muscles (the gastrocnemius and soleus) is that they are seldom strengthened throughout their full range of motion. If you neglect proper calf strengthening or place the calf in a shortened position (by wearing high heels, for example), you will weaken your Achilles tendon.[1] This tendon connects the calf muscles to the heel bone and accounts for up to 11% of all running injuries.[1]

Research indicates that heel drops are an essential component of proper calf strengthening.[2] However, this component tends to be neglected during calf raises. Whether you wish to improve your calf aesthetics or minimize your risk of Achilles tendon problems, the following chapter provides help. You will learn proper calf strengthening using the standing and seated calf machines. But don't worry if you do not have access to a machine—you can simply use a stair or ledge.

EQUIPMENT OPTIONS

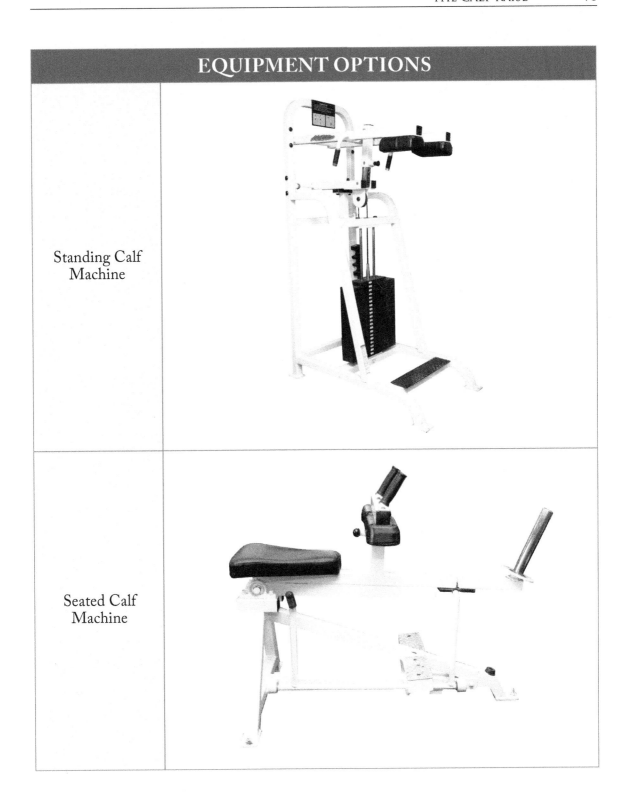

Standing Calf
Machine

Seated Calf
Machine

KEY POINTS FOR A SAFE AND EFFECTIVE CALF RAISE

1. **Foot position**

   Begin with your heels below your toes (as far as possible) to obtain a full range of motion and optimize the stretch in your Achilles tendon.

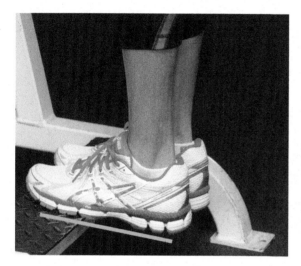
Correct

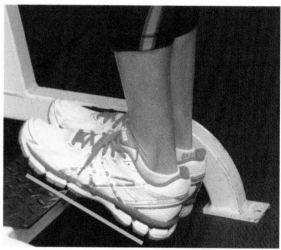
Correct (preferred)

Weight-Training Tip

The calf raise appears relatively simple,
but if you want results, do not neglect this exercise.

MASTER TECHNIQUE: STANDING CALF RAISE

The standing calf machine is the recommended equipment of choice for the calf raise. It allows a full range of motion and enables you to use more weight than in a seated position.

1. Start

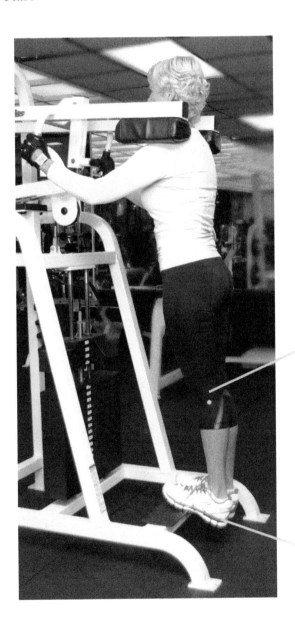

Knee position
Keep your knees locked.

Foot position
Drop your heels below your toes.

2. **Finish**

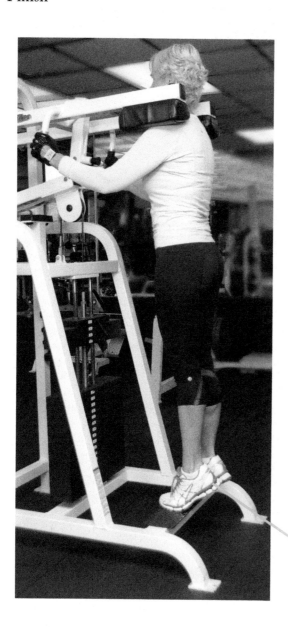

Foot position

Raise your heels as high as possible.

SEATED CALF RAISE

You can not use as much weight with the seated calf machine as the standing one. Specifically, bending your knees disengages a portion of your calf (the gastrocnemius).[3] Therefore, results come slower.

1. **Start**

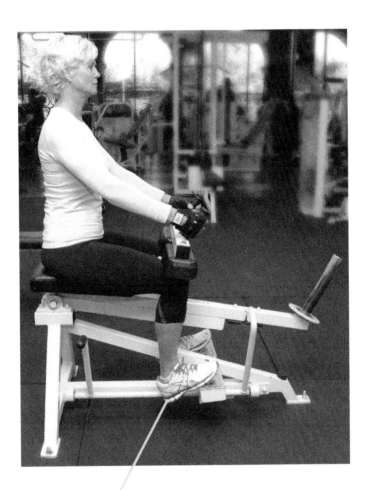

Foot position

Drop your heels below your toes.

2. Finish

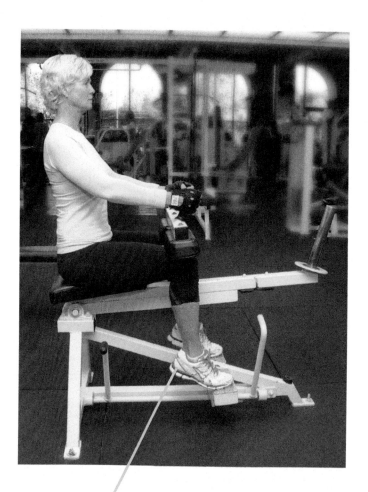

Foot position

Raise your heels as high
as possible.

SECTION III

BACK

The Lat Pulldown

The lat pulldown gives you the perfect V. In other words,
it makes the upper portion of your back larger than the middle or lower.

THE LAT PULLDOWN ("LAT" IS SHORT for the latissimus dorsi, the widest muscle of the back) is a standard back exercise that requires you to pull weights (attached to a machine) from above your head to your chest.

This chapter explains why you should *never* pull the weight behind your head, as well as the differences in handgrip variations.

EQUIPMENT OPTIONS

Lat Pulldown
Machine
+
Handgrip Choice

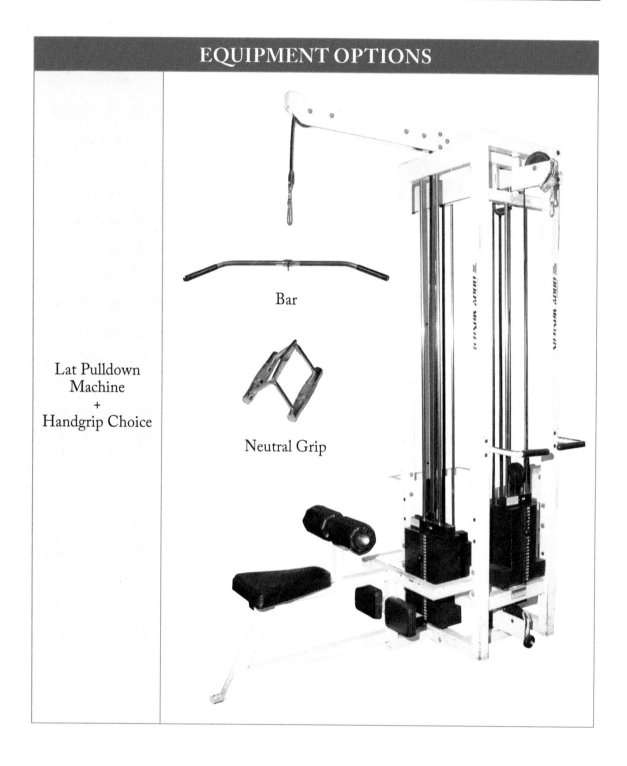

Bar

Neutral Grip

KEY POINTS FOR A SAFE
AND EFFECTIVE LAT PULLDOWN

1. Handgrip

Use a palm-down grip. A neutral grip (thumbs on top—a position that places your palms facing inward) or a palm-up grip can be used, but they are less effective for strengthening your lats.[1,2]

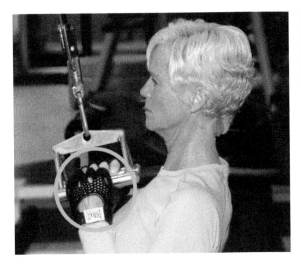

Correct (neutral)

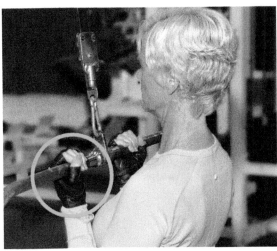

Correct (palm up)

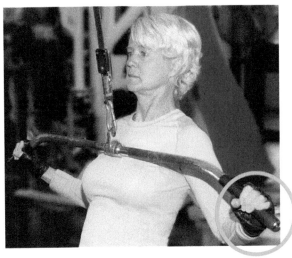

Correct (preferred) (palm down)

2. Weight position

Never pull the bar behind your head. There's no activity or sport where you pull anything behind your head! And for a good reason: performing this exercise behind your head can cause irreparable damage to your rotator cuff (group of muscles and tendons that protects and stabilizes the shoulder joint and facilitates proper shoulder function) and neck, and can even result in upper extremity paralysis.[1,3]

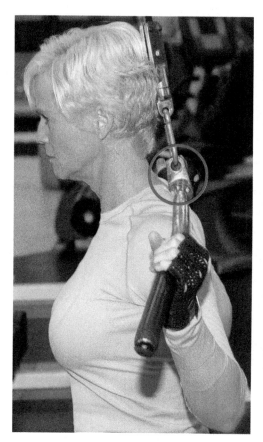

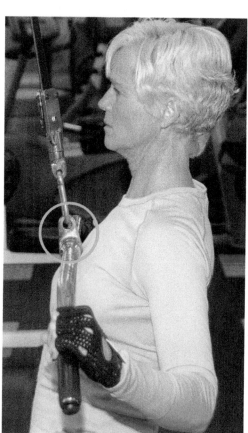

Incorrect   Correct

3. Back position

Lean your torso slightly back to minimize the strain on your low back.

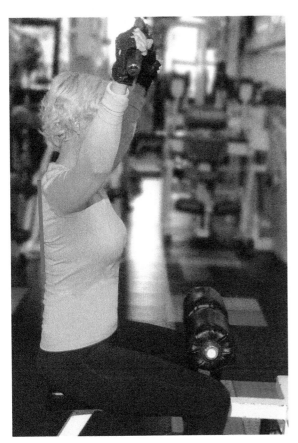
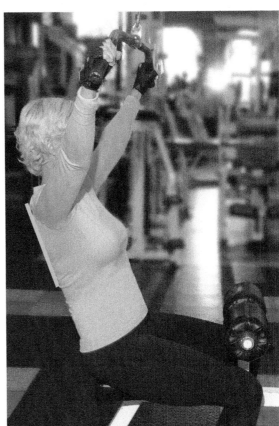

Incorrect   Correct

MASTER TECHNIQUE: PALM-DOWN LAT PULLDOWN

The lat pulldown is most effective for lat development when your hands are placed palm down. With this type of orientation, there's no difference between a shoulder-width and wider grip. Select your preference.[2]

1. Start

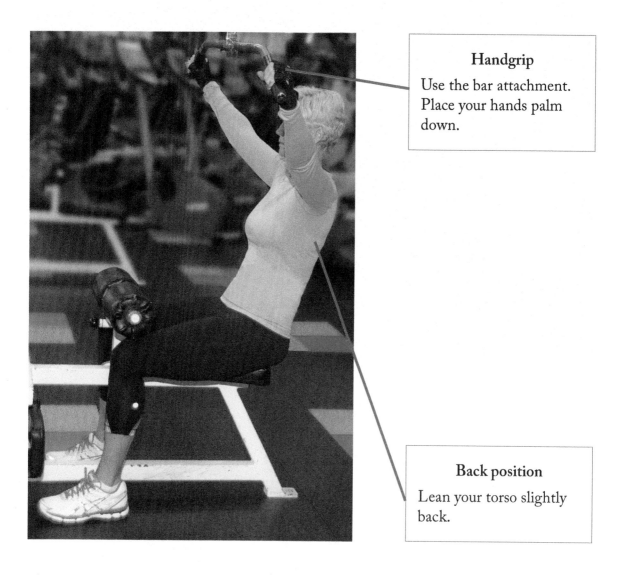

Handgrip
Use the bar attachment. Place your hands palm down.

Back position
Lean your torso slightly back.

2. Finish

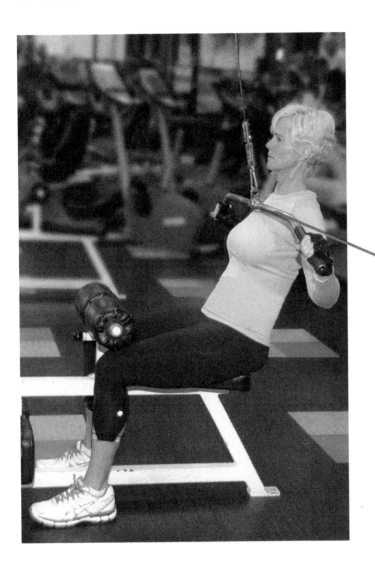

Weight position

Pull the bar to your chest—*never* behind your head.

THE ROW

*Generally, the lat pulldown is preferable to the row
for back strengthening. However, the row does offer variety.*

THE ROW EMPHASIZES DIFFERENT REGIONS OF your back than the lat pulldown does—specifically the middle trapezius and rhomboids (muscles that help pull your shoulders back),[1] which makes it good for postural enhancement.

There are multiple variations, but for simplicity we categorize rowing exercises into machine rows and dumbbell rows. In this chapter, we outline the benefits of each, along with the best choice of equipment.

EQUIPMENT OPTIONS

Seated Machine Row	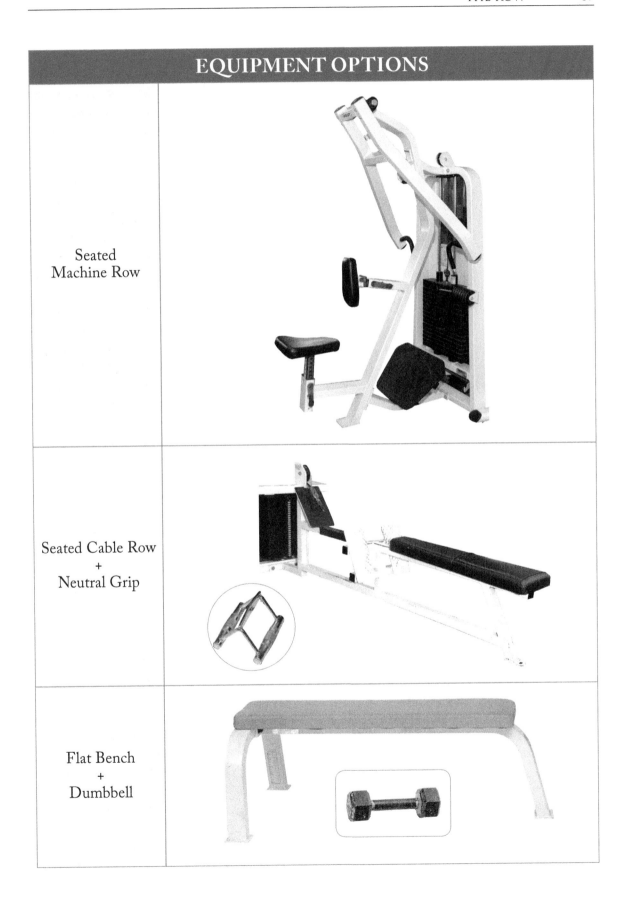
Seated Cable Row + Neutral Grip	
Flat Bench + Dumbbell	

KEY POINTS FOR A SAFE AND EFFECTIVE ROW

1. Exercises to be avoided

Avoid performing freestanding bent-over rows because such exercises place high loads on your lumbar spine.[2]

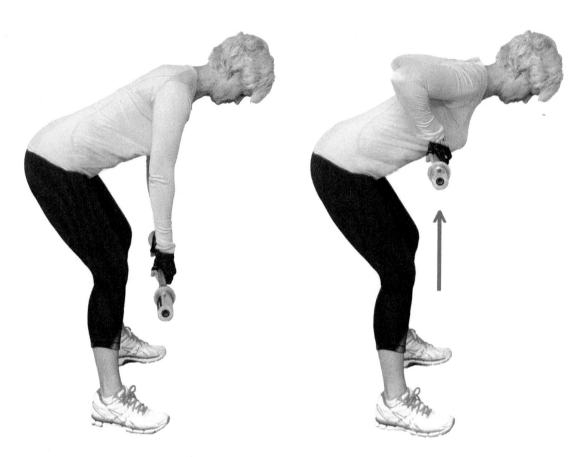

Freestanding Bent-over Row (to be avoided)

Weight-Training Tip

Although it is impossible for us to demonstrate all the weight-training exercises that will predispose you to injury, we hope that if you study this book, you will acquire the ability to determine what is safe and what is not.

---

2. Head position (for the dumbbell row)

Keep your head down to avoid neck strain.

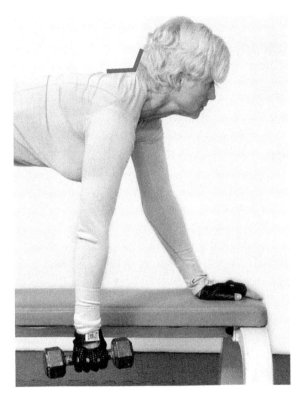
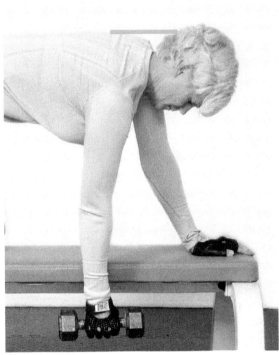

Incorrect   Correct

3. Handgrip

Use a neutral grip (thumbs on top—a grip that places your palms facing inward). A palm-down grip can lead to shoulder impingement, particularly when your elbows are maintained at shoulder height.[3]

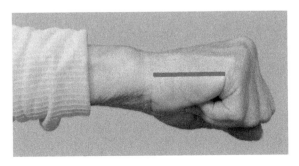
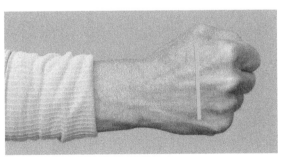

Incorrect (palm down)   Correct (neutral)

4. **Back position**

   Avoid rounding your back. Rounding your back places your low back in a vulnerable position.

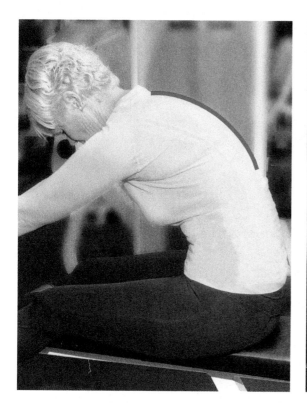 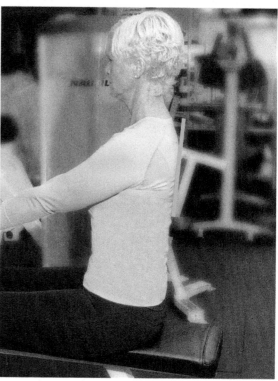

Incorrect   Correct

Weight-Training Tip

*The back region is the most vulnerable to injury during the row.
As such, pay particular attention to your posture during any row exercise.*

MASTER TECHNIQUE: MACHINE ROW

The primary benefit of the machine row is that it hastens development of your back. We recommend machines that provide stabilization, such as those shown below, to maintain proper form.

Variation 1: Seated Machine Row

The main benefit of the seated machine row is that it facilities maintenance of proper back positioning.

1. **Start**

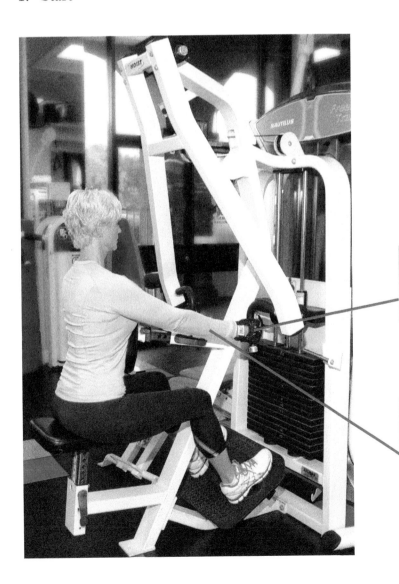

Handgrip
Use a neutral grip.

Arm position
Allow your arms to be pulled completely forward for the full range of motion. Adjust the seat if necessary.

2. Finish

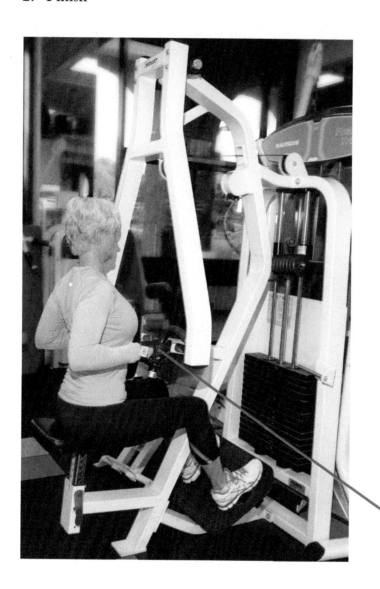

Weight position

Pull the weight back as far as possible.

Variation 2: Seated Cable Row

The seated cable row can be performed using a variety of handgrips. We advise any neutral grip attachment that places your thumbs on top (with palms facing inward, as shown)—it's safer for your shoulders.

1. **Start**

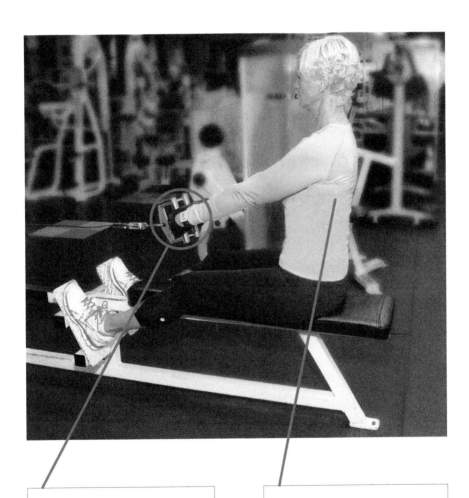

Handgrip

Use a neutral grip attachment.

Back position

Keep good posture. A slightly backward lean is natural.

2. Finish

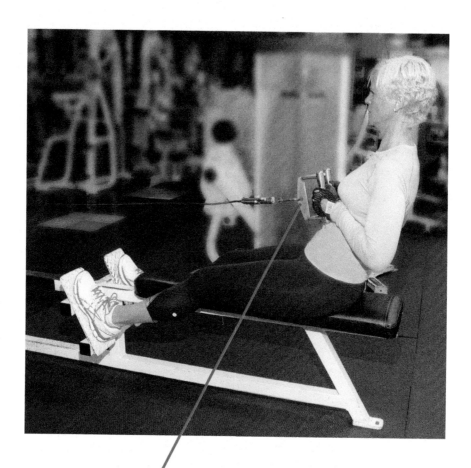

Weight position

Pull the weight to your lower chest.

DUMBBELL ROW

The primary benefit of the dumbbell row is that it allows for more range of motion. We recommend a bench for stabilization.

1. **Start**

Back position

Keep your back flat. *Avoid* arching.

Head position

Keep your head down to avoid neck strain.

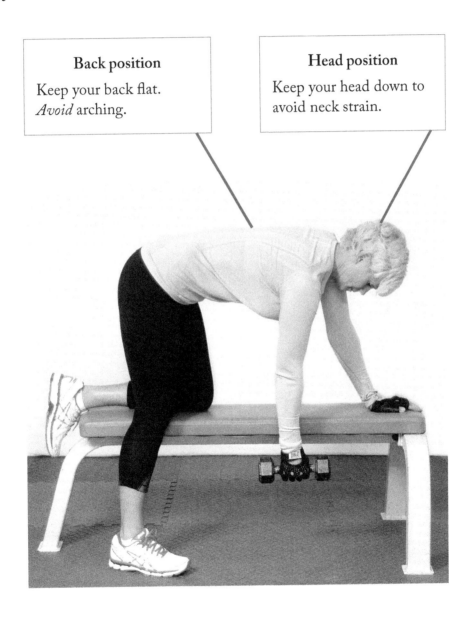

2. Finish

Weight position

Pull the dumbbell to your underarm for the full range of motion.

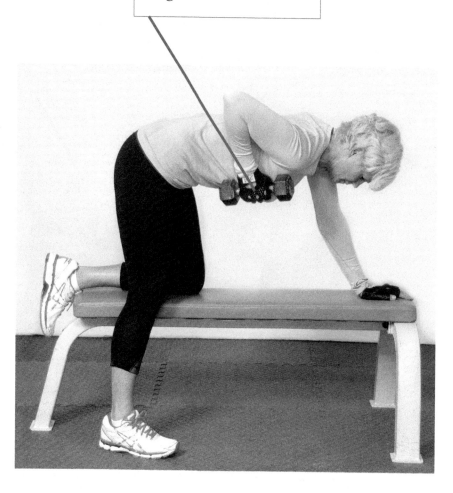

THE REVERSE FLY

The reverse fly targets the region between your shoulder blades and is one of the most important, if not the most important, postural exercises.

T HE REVERSE FLY EMPHASIZES YOUR BACK postural muscles (such as the middle trapezius and rhomboids) to a greater extent than the row, and so the exercise is essential to your back routine.[1] To ensure its effectiveness, it is imperative that you obtain the full range of motion, and to achieve this a low weight is a must.

In this chapter, we show you three ways of performing the reverse fly: the cable system, the reverse fly machine, and dumbbells.

EQUIPMENT OPTIONS

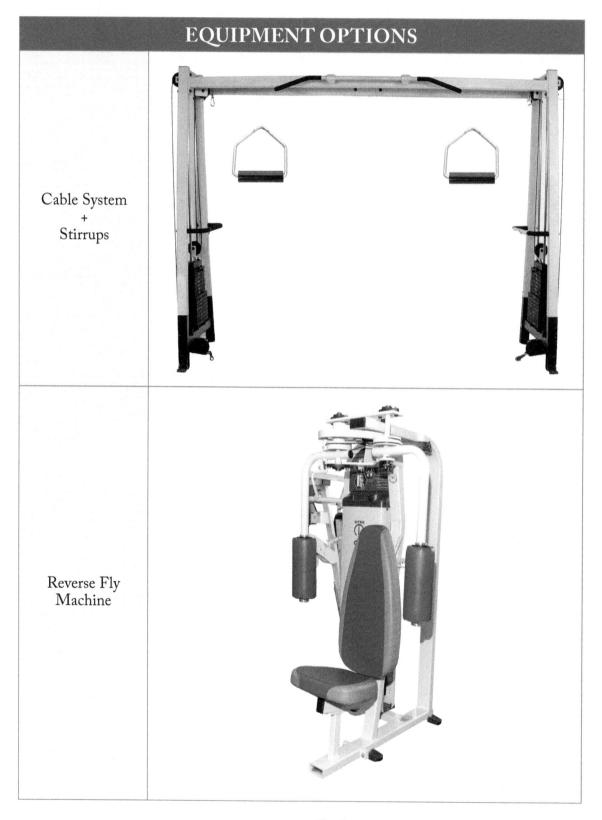

Cable System
+
Stirrups

Reverse Fly
Machine

Equipment options continue on the next page.

Dumbbells	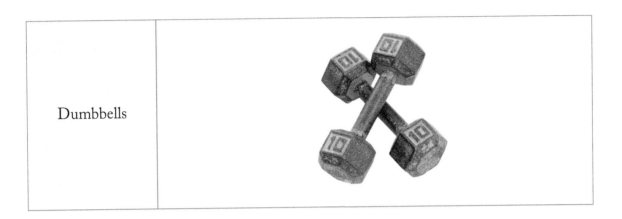

Weight-Training Tip

As we mentioned earlier, low weight is a must for this exercise to be effective. Therefore, any of the exercises in this chapter can be performed without the use of any weight. Choose your favorite method and execute the motion consistently (even daily) to achieve results.

KEY POINTS FOR A SAFE AND EFFECTIVE REVERSE FLY

1. Arm position

To truly benefit from this exercise, you *must* obtain a complete range of motion. This requires you to keep your elbows below your shoulders when pulling your arms back—the exact height of your arms in relation to your shoulders will vary with the type of reverse fly. Additionally, maintaining your elbows below shoulder level helps avoid shoulder impingement.[2]

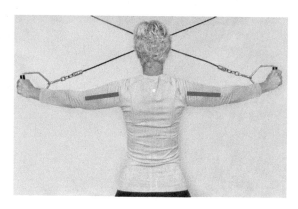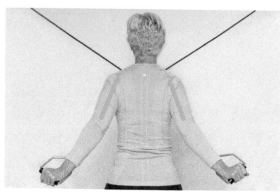

Incorrect	Correct

2. Back position

Keep your shoulders back. Rounding your shoulders strains the muscles of your back and increases the chance of injury. This is relevant to any movement but is particularly important when your torso is forward (as for the dumbbell reverse fly).

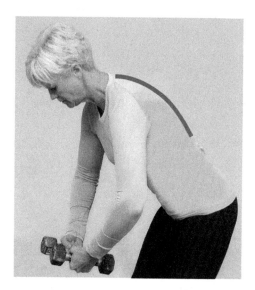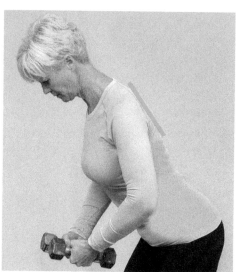

Incorrect	Correct

MASTER TECHNIQUE: CABLE REVERSE FLY

The cable reverse fly is the most beneficial for targeting the region between your shoulder blades.

1. Start

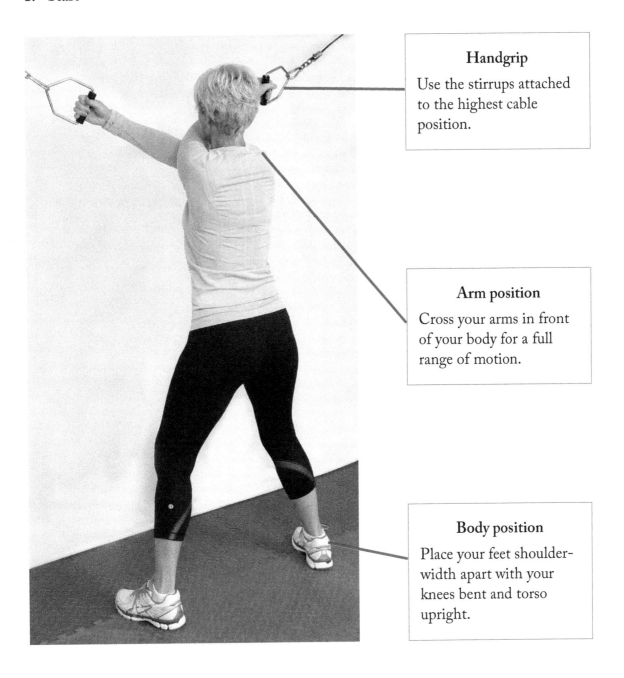

Handgrip
Use the stirrups attached to the highest cable position.

Arm position
Cross your arms in front of your body for a full range of motion.

Body position
Place your feet shoulder-width apart with your knees bent and torso upright.

2. Finish

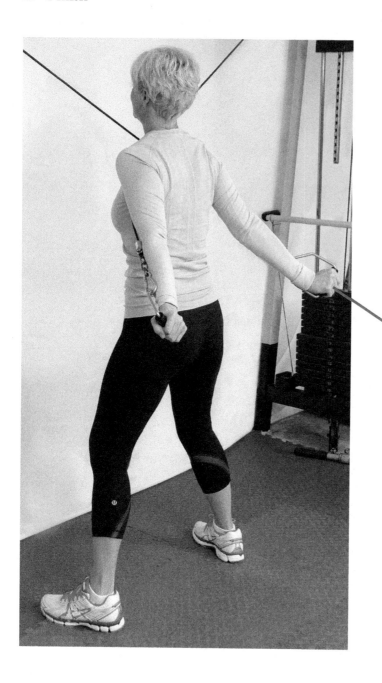

Arm position

Pull your arms back as far as possible. Keep your elbows below your shoulders.

MACHINE REVERSE FLY

The machine reverse fly makes attaining proper form easier but is the least effective for targeting the muscles between your shoulders blades, as the range of motion tends to be limited. Depending on the machine's design, you may need to place your elbows on the pads (as shown) rather than the gripping handles.

1. Start

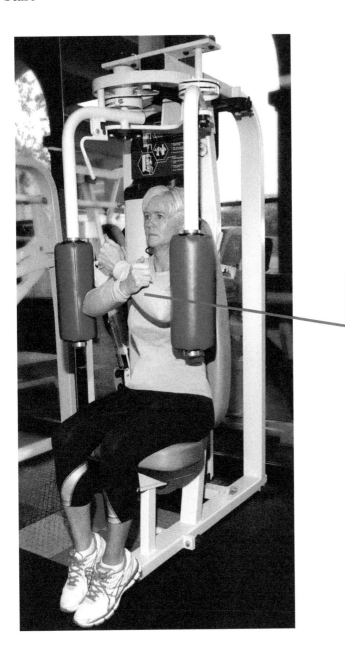

Arm position

Cross your arms in front of your body for a full range of motion.

2. Finish

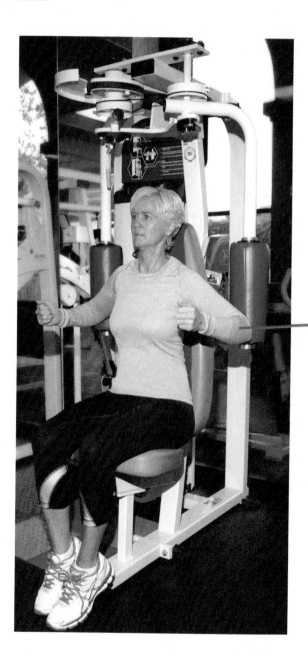

Arm position

Pull your arms back as far as possible. Keep your elbows slightly bent and below your shoulders.

DUMBBELL REVERSE FLY

You can perform the dumbbell reverse fly using a variety of techniques. However, the variation shown is the one we prefer. Remember, this is a back move. Therefore, if you don't feel activity in your back, your arms are likely too far forward at the finish.

1. **Start**

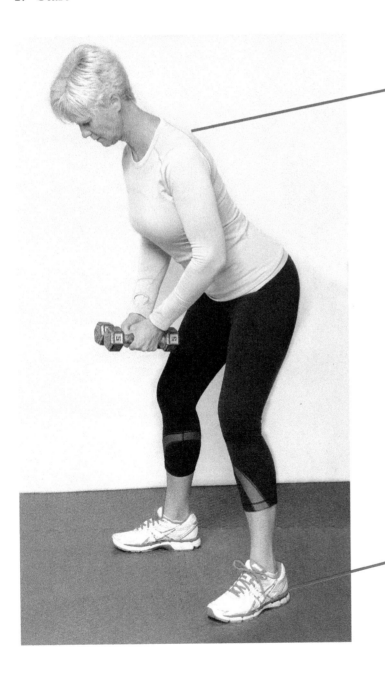

Back position

Keep your shoulders back. *Avoid* rounding your shoulders.

Body position

Place your feet shoulder-width apart with your knees bent and torso slightly forward.

2. Finish

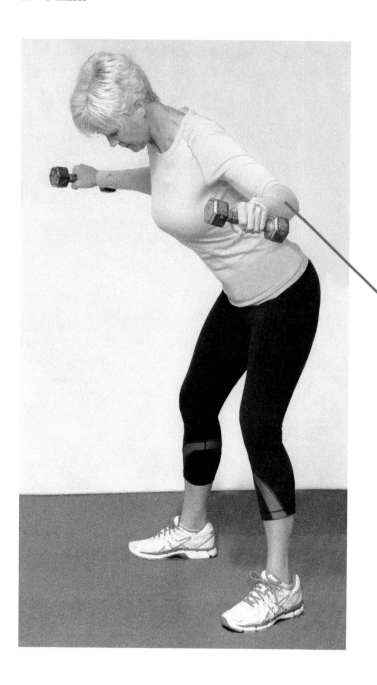

Arm position

Raise your arms up and back until your forearms are horizontal to the floor. Keep your elbows slightly bent and below your shoulders.

THE LOW-BACK EXTENSION

Low-back exercises are only one component of core strengthening.

LOW-BACK EXERCISES ARE COMMONLY RECOMMENDED to enhance low-back strength. However, the muscles of the low back are seldom weak, and so it is not surprising that there is little relation between low-back strength and the risk of low-back injury.[1,2,3] Then why, you may ask, do up to 85% of adults at some point in their life suffer from low-back pain?[4]

The answer is not simple, but there are a few general reasons: Glute weakness exacerbates back troubles; in other words, weakness at the hip results in compensation at the back.[2,5] Also, improper form during any kind of activity can easily result in low-back injury. In fact, the low back sustains the highest number of injuries in competitive lifters (23%), closely followed by the knees and shoulders.[6] And, surprisingly, there are machines supposedly designed for low-back strengthening that are extremely dangerous (as we elucidate in the following pages).

Nonetheless, low-back exercises can promote low-back health. In this chapter, we demonstrate a key low-back exercise that is quite enjoyable. We should also point out, however, that the integrity of *all* the muscles surrounding the low back (termed the "core") are essential for the prevention of low-back pain. We deal with the core in detail in Section VII.

EQUIPMENT OPTIONS

Exercise Mat	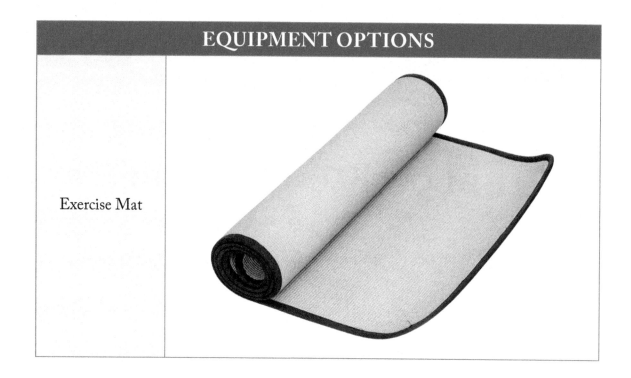

Weight-Training Tip

An exercise mat is not essential for this exercise, though it can be comfortable. In fact, any surface can be used (even your bed) as long as it is firm.

KEY POINTS FOR A SAFE AND EFFECTIVE LOW-BACK EXTENSION

1. **Equipment to be avoided**

   Avoid the Roman chair (pictured on this page—a bench that locks your feet so you can lift your body weight with your low back). Performing back extensions using this piece of equipment can result in serious back injury (such as disc herniation).[2]

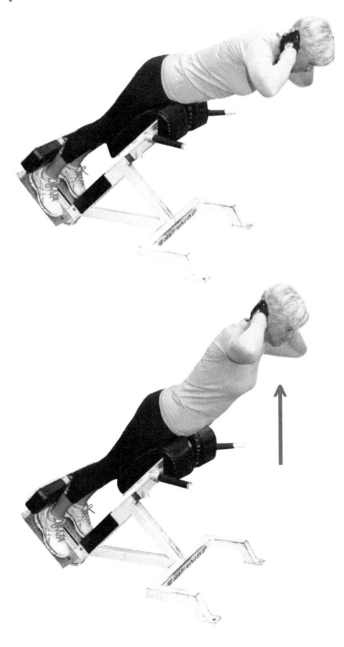

Back Extensions Using Roman Chair (to be avoided)

2. Hip position (for the press-up)

Keep your hips flush with the ground to minimize stress on your low back. Placing your hands in front of your body (and not directly under) will help. If you experience any discomfort in your low back, your hands are too far back!

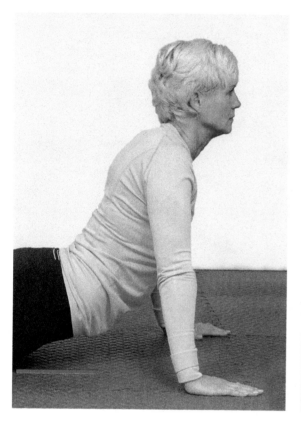

Incorrect

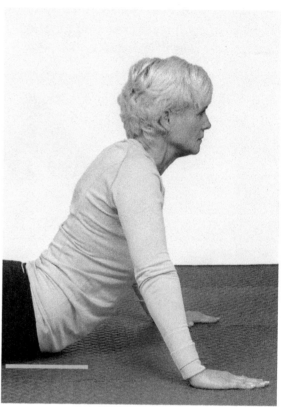

Correct

MASTER TECHNIQUE: PRESS-UP

The press-up is one of the best exercises for your low back. Research indicates that the press-up helps prevent and relieve low-back pain.[7, 8] Considering that most activities place your spine in a flexed or forward position (do you slouch often?), you may find this exercise challenging at first.

Stage 1

Before beginning the press-up exercise, make sure you can comfortably perform the "sphinx" position shown.

1. Start and Finish

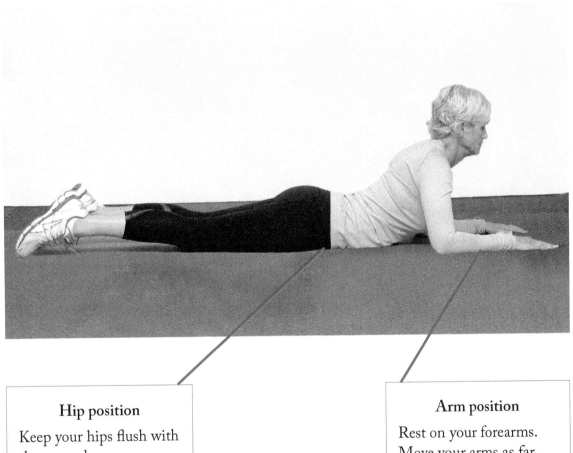

Hip position

Keep your hips flush with the ground.

Arm position

Rest on your forearms. Move your arms as far forward as needed so you are comfortable.

Stage 2

Once you are comfortable with the "sphinx" position, you are ready to try the press-up. Aim to perform this move comfortably with repetitions. Endurance (more repetitions at low resistance) rather than strength (fewer repetitions at high resistance) has the most influence on the integrity and health of your low back.[2, 3]

1. Start

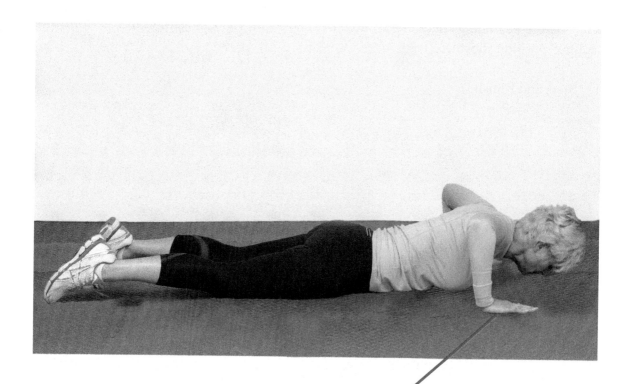

Hand position

Place your hands near your shoulders.

2. Finish

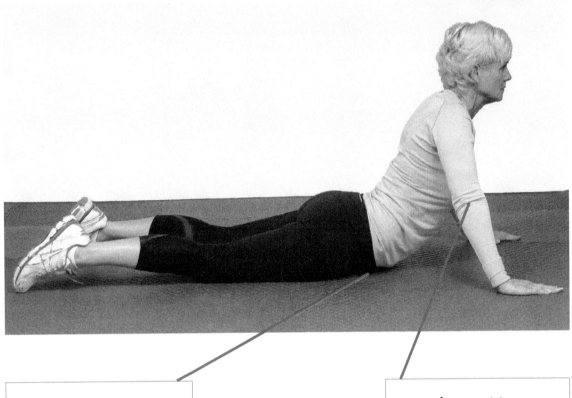

Hip position

Keep your hips flush with the ground.

Arm position

Straighten your elbows. Keep your hands in front of your shoulders to avoid lifting your hips (and thereby straining your low back).

SECTION IV

CHEST

THE BENCH PRESS

The bench press has everything to do with appearance but little to do with upper-body strength.

THE BENCH PRESS IS ONE OF the most, if not the most, popular upper-body exercises. The amount of weight an individual can "bench" is often used as a way to evaluate upper-body strength. Even the National Football League (NFL) uses the bench press to screen potential players, though the ability of bench press strength to predict player performance remains questionable.[1]

It is possible to bench up to 5 times your body weight when lying flat, but while standing, individuals can only push up to half their body weight.[2,3] So you can see that the bench press is not a real indicator of functional upper-body strength.

Bench pressing is useful for increasing the size and appearance of your chest, but be aware that the exercise is also a primary cause of shoulder injury.[3-6] Fortunately, in this chapter, we focus on the proper, injury-free method of bench pressing so you may better isolate your chest and avoid shoulder injury. You will learn why arm placement is key for injury prevention and the difference between using a flat bench and an incline bench.

EQUIPMENT OPTIONS

Bench Choice	Weight Choice

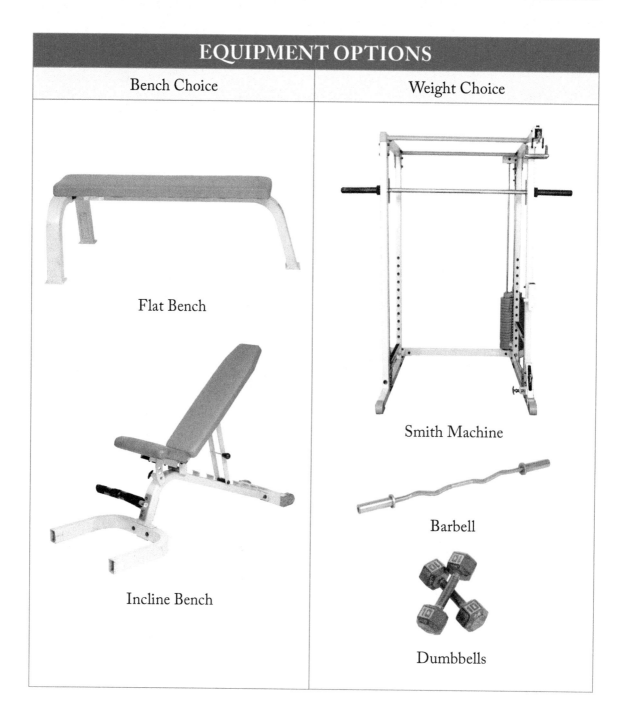

Flat Bench

Incline Bench

Smith Machine

Barbell

Dumbbells

KEY POINTS FOR A SAFE
AND EFFECTIVE BENCH PRESS

1. Arm position

Keep the angle between your torso and upper arms slightly below 90°. This keeps your elbows below shoulder level throughout the exercise, which reduces irritation to shoulder structures such as the rotator cuff and bursa.[5]

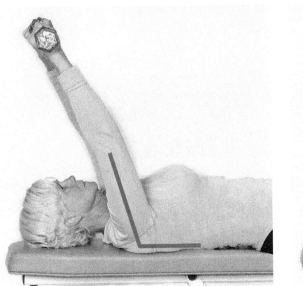

Incorrect

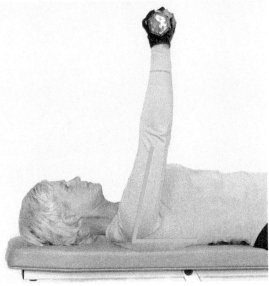

Correct

Weight-Training Tip

Maintaining your elbows below shoulder level is always achievable when using a flat bench (as shown above). Conversely, maintaining your elbows below shoulder levels is not always possible when using an incline bench; therefore, the incline bench press may be troublesome for those with shoulder problems.[5, 7] Regardless of the type of bench you choose, you will minimize your risk of injury if you follow the Key Points outlined in this chapter.

Avoid flaring your elbows, as that increases the risk of shoulder injury. Your elbows should be no wider than 45°.[7, 8] Generally, wider handgrips increase elbow flaring. Although wider handgrips may enhance chest activation (notably to the pectoralis major, which is the largest and most visible chest muscle),[9] any potential benefit is not worth the increased injury risk.

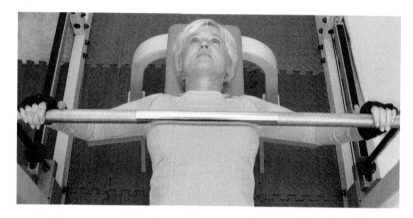

Incorrect

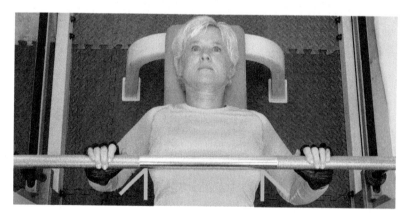

Correct

2. Weight position

If you're using the flat bench, the weight should hit your middle chest (directly if using a barbell or Smith machine, as shown, or on the sides if using dumbbells).

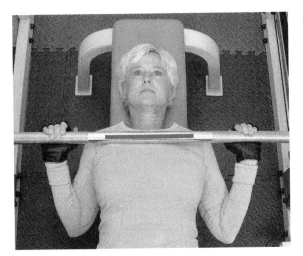
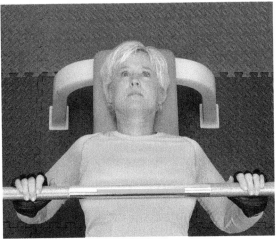

Incorrect   Correct

If you're using the incline bench, the weight should hit slightly above the middle of your chest (directly if using a barbell or Smith machine, as shown, or on the sides if using dumbbells).

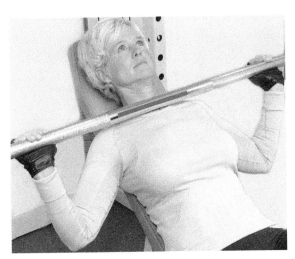
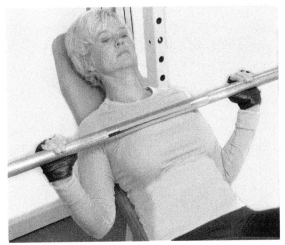

Incorrect   Correct

3. **Back position (when using a flat bench)**
    Avoid arching your low back excessively—it should maintain its natural position (slightly curved). Arching your low back excessively (generally to compensate for the use of too much weight) can injure it.

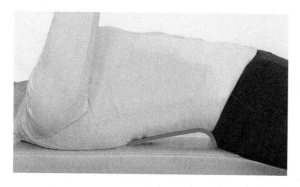 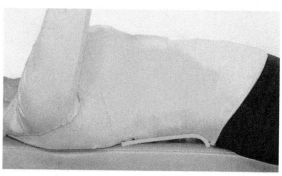

Incorrect   Correct

4. **Bench position**
    The position of the bench determines the area of your chest activated. The flat bench targets the middle to lower portion. The incline bench targets the upper portion. Position the bench at approximately 45° from horizontal for the greatest benefit.[10]

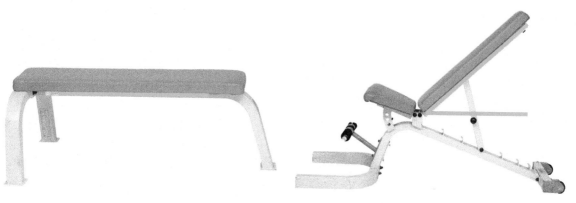

Flat Bench   Incline Bench

MASTER TECHNIQUE: FLAT BENCH PRESS

The flat bench is the recommended equipment of choice, as it targets the largest area of your chest.

Variation 1: Flat Bench Press (Using Barbell or Smith Machine)

The flat bench with a barbell tends to result in greater muscle activity.[11] However, the Smith machine, or any machine that guides the bar, eliminates human error and that's why we prefer it.

1. **Start**

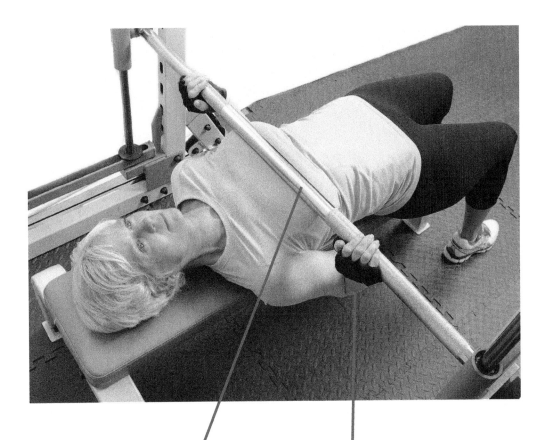

Weight position

Let the bar hit the middle of your chest.

Arm position

Keep your elbows close to your body.

2. **Finish**

Weight position

Push the bar upward.

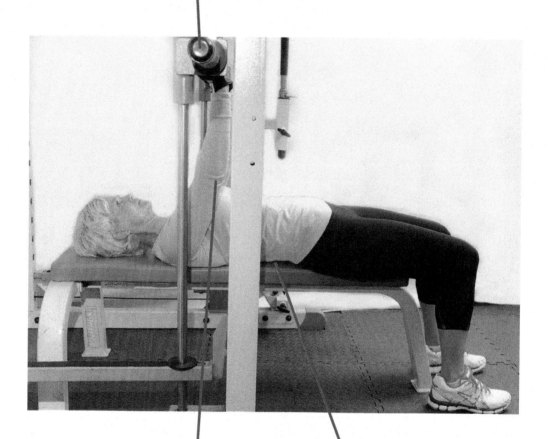

Arm position

Keep the angle between your torso and upper arms slightly below 90°.

Back position

Keep your low back in its natural position. *Avoid* arching excessively.

Variation 2: Flat Bench Press (Using Dumbbells)

Dumbbells are more effective in shaping and building your chest than a bar. The bar stops at the level of your chest, preventing the full range of motion. However, the use of a fuller range of motion can be dangerous if done improperly—remember, *avoid* elbow flaring![8]

1. **Start**

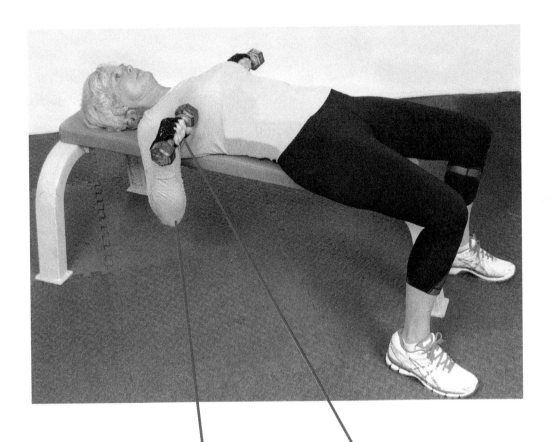

Arm position

Keep your elbows close to your body.

Weight position

Bring the dumbbells to the side of your middle chest.

2. Finish

Weight position

Push the dumbbells upward.

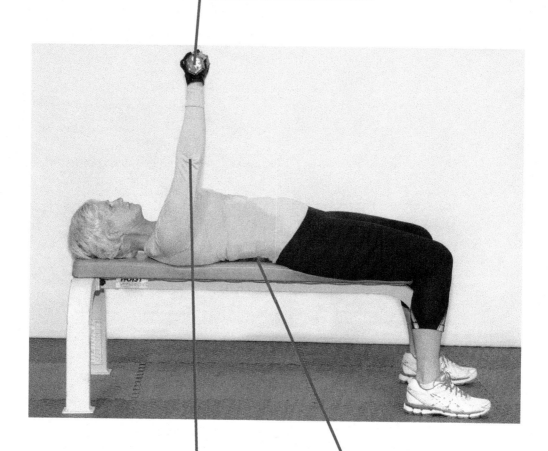

Arm position

Keep the angle between your torso and upper arms slightly below 90°.

Back position

Keep your low back in its natural position. *Avoid* arching excessively.

INCLINE BENCH PRESS

The incline bench press enhances development of your upper chest.

Variation 1: Incline Bench Press (Using Barbell or Smith Machine)

As with the flat bench press, we prefer the Smith machine over a barbell for safety reasons. But when using the Smith machine (or a barbell, if you so choose), please note the angle between your upper arms and torso will be slightly above 90°. If this is a concern, you can use the dumbbell version instead.

1. **Start**

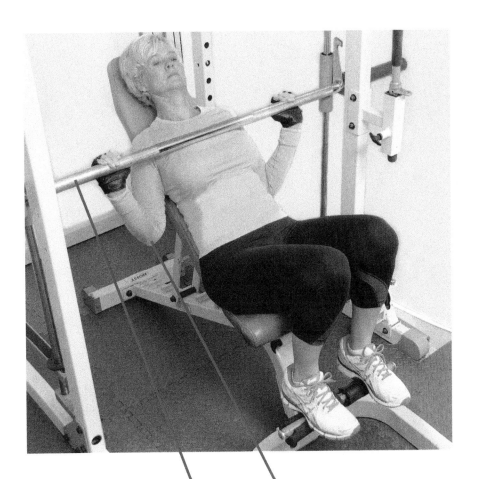

Weight position

Let the bar hit just above the middle of your chest.

Arm position

Keep your elbows close to your body.

2. Finish

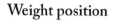

Weight position

Push the bar upward.

Arm position

Keep the angle between your torso and upper arms as close to 90° as possible.

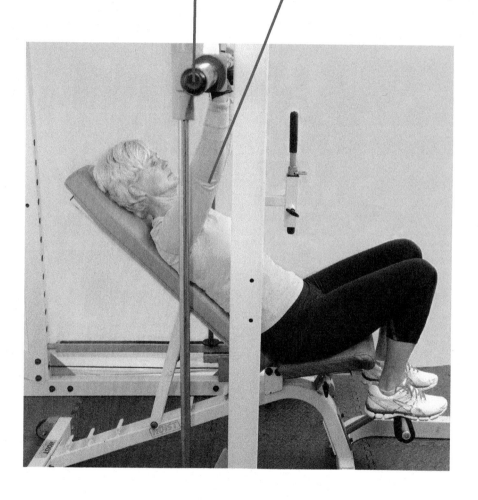

Variation 2: Incline Bench Press (Using Dumbbells)

Dumbbells enable a fuller range of motion than a bar, making them the equipment of choice by professionals for chest strengthening.

1. **Start**

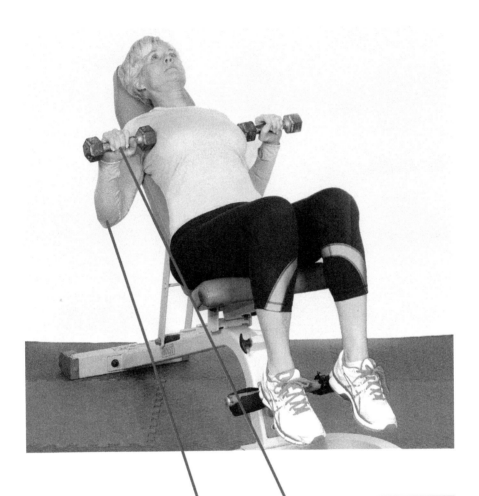

Arm position

Keep your elbows close to your body.

Weight position

Bring the dumbbells to your side, slightly above the middle of your chest.

2. Finish

Arm position

Ideally, keep the angle between your torso and upper arms slightly below 90°.

Weight position

Push the dumbbells upward.

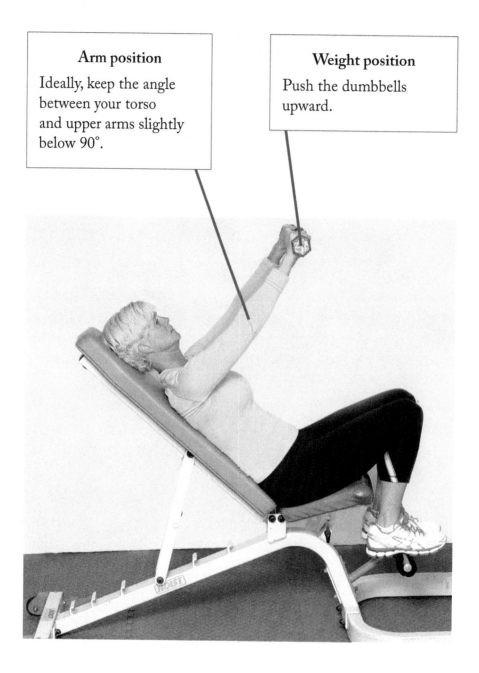

14

THE CHEST FLY

It is commonly believed that bench presses are optimal for chest development when in fact they are not. Chest flies are far superior.

ALTHOUGH BENCH PRESSES ALLOW YOU TO use more weight, chest flies are essential for proper chest development. Chest flies engage a larger region of your chest by stretching the muscle throughout its entire length. However, if you perform them improperly, they can increase the likelihood of shoulder troubles.[1]

Therefore, in this chapter we show you the proper chest fly technique (*without* compromising the integrity of the shoulder complex) using dumbbells, a cable system, and the chest fly machine.

EQUIPMENT OPTIONS

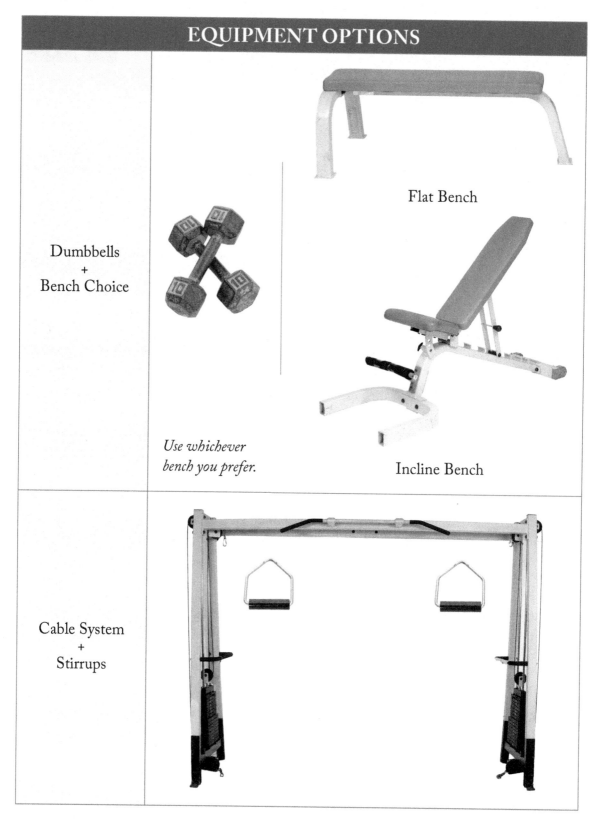

Dumbbells
+
Bench Choice

Flat Bench

Use whichever bench you prefer.

Incline Bench

Cable System
+
Stirrups

Equipment options continue on the next page.

Chest Fly
Machine

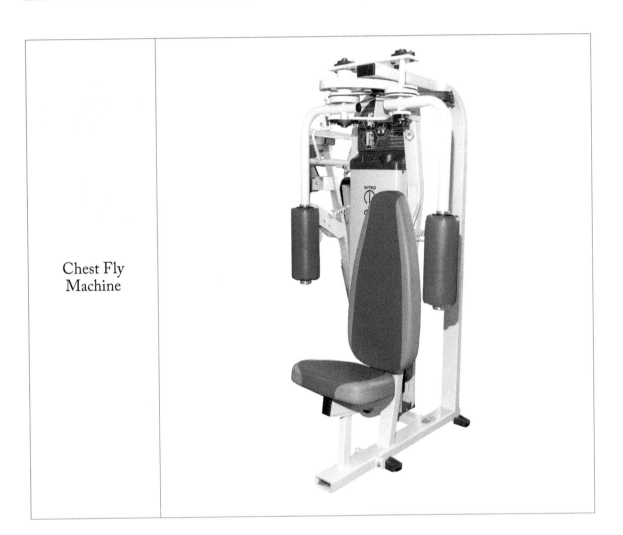

KEY POINTS FOR A SAFE
AND EFFECTIVE CHEST FLY

1. Handgrip

Use a neutral grip (thumbs on top—a grip that places your hands facing inward). A palm-down grip can lead to shoulder impingement, particularly when your elbows are kept at shoulder height.[2]

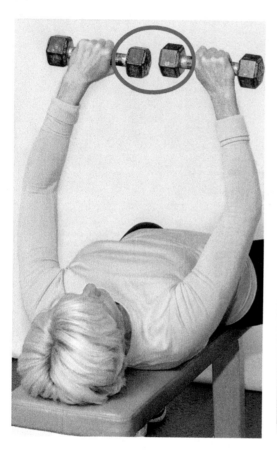

Incorrect

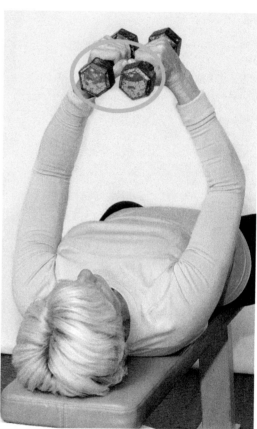

Correct

2. Arm position

Ideally, keep the angle between your torso and upper arms slightly below 90° (that is, your elbows below shoulder level) to reduce the risk of shoulder injury.[2] This is easiest to do when using a flat bench. If using an incline bench (shown below), the angle between your upper arms and torso will be approximately 90° (as demonstrated in the "Correct" picture); for this it is particularly important to ensure your handgrip is proper.

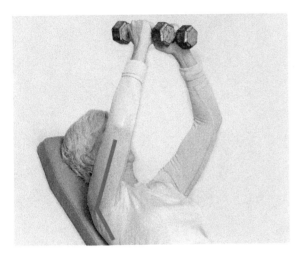

Incorrect

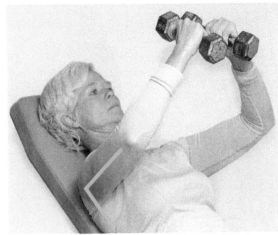

Correct

Keep your elbows slightly bent. Flattening your elbows can injure your shoulders and elbows.

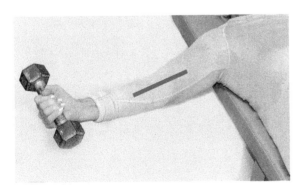

Incorrect

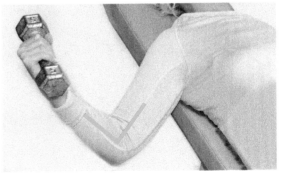

Correct

Open your arms wide (in an arc, as if hugging a barrel). Using too narrow an arc allows your elbows to move excessively past your shoulders, which increases the risk of injury for some (and is less effective). If you have a previous shoulder injury, you may need to restrict your range of motion.[2]

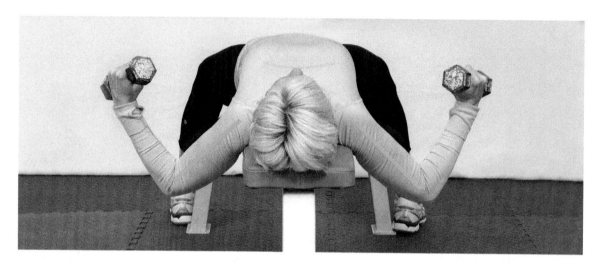

Correct

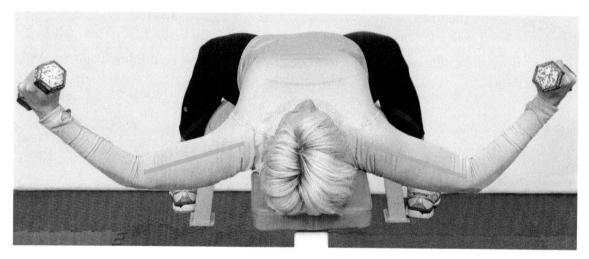

Correct (preferred)

If you are using a chest fly machine, maintain a horizontal forearm—placing your forearms vertical can lead to decreased shoulder stability and eventual dislocation.[1]

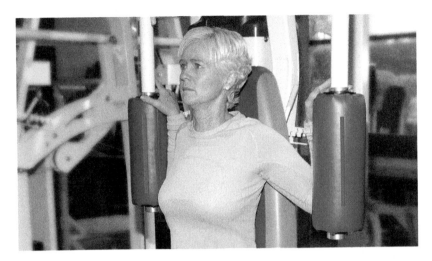

Incorrect

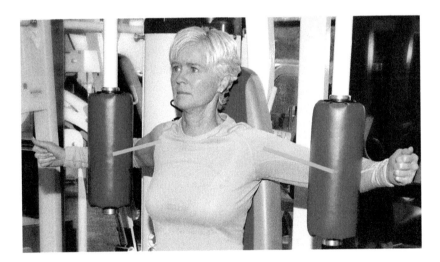

Correct

3. Back position (for the standing cable chest fly)

Keep your back flat—if you keep your shoulders back, this should occur naturally. Rounding your back increases the chance of injury, particularly to your low back.

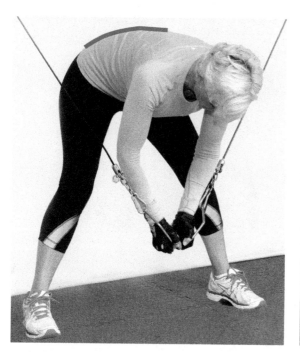

Incorrect

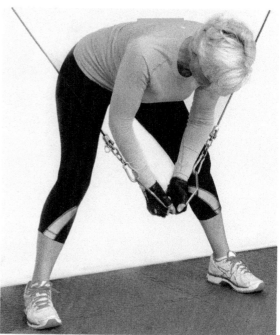

Correct

4. Bench position

The position of the bench determines the area of your chest that's activated. The flat bench targets the middle to lower portion. The incline bench targets the upper portion. Position the bench at approximately 45° from horizontal for the greatest benefit.

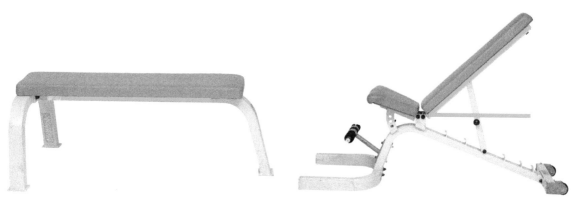

Flat Bench

Incline Bench

MASTER TECHNIQUE: FLAT BENCH CHEST FLY

The flat bench is the recommended equipment of choice, as it targets the largest area of your chest.

1. Start

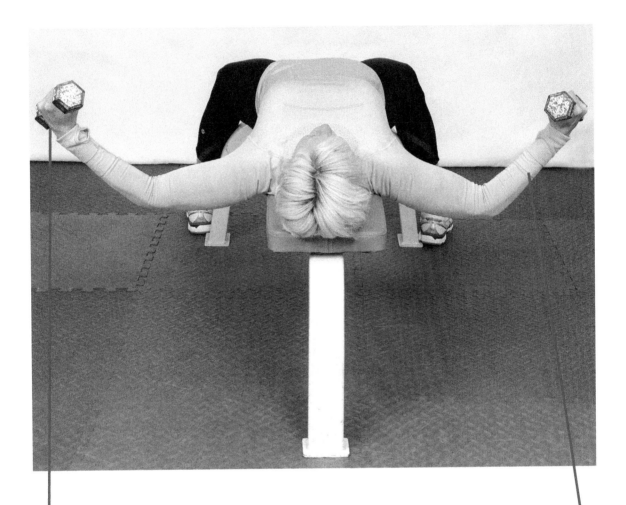

Handgrip

Use a neutral grip.

Arm position

Open your arms wide. Keep your elbows slightly bent.

2. Finish

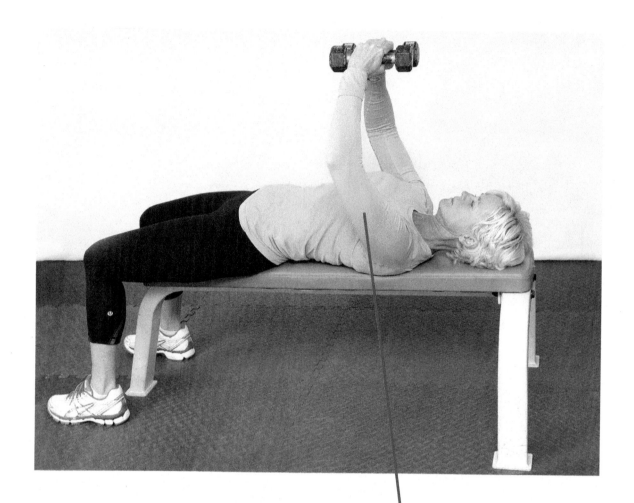

Arm position

Move your arms in an arc as if hugging a barrel. Keep the angle between your torso and upper arms slightly below 90°.

INCLINE BENCH CHEST FLY

The incline bench chest fly enhances development of your upper chest. Remember that this variation makes it difficult to maintain the angle between your upper arms and torso below 90°, so pay careful attention to your handgrip.

1. **Start**

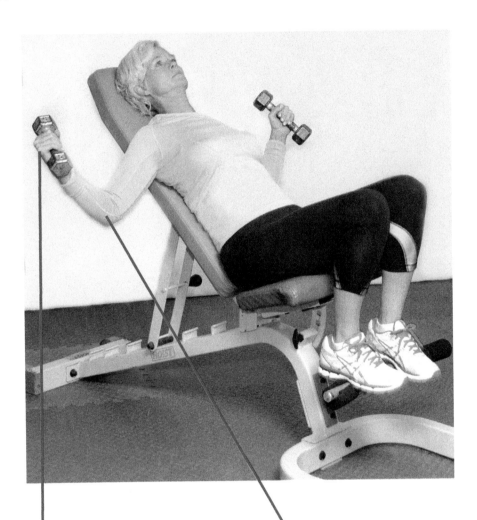

Handgrip

Use a neutral grip.

Arm position

Open your arms wide. Keep your elbows slightly bent.

2. Finish

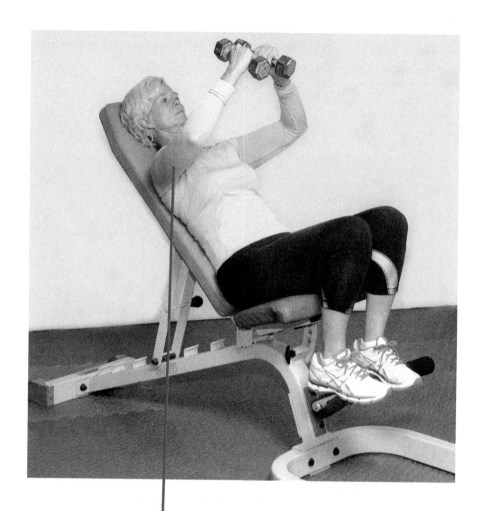

Arm position

Move your arms in an
arc as if hugging a
barrel. Ideally, keep the angle
between your torso and
upper arms slightly
below 90°.

STANDING CABLE CHEST FLY

This move is a variation of the preceding flat bench dumbbell version.

1. **Start**

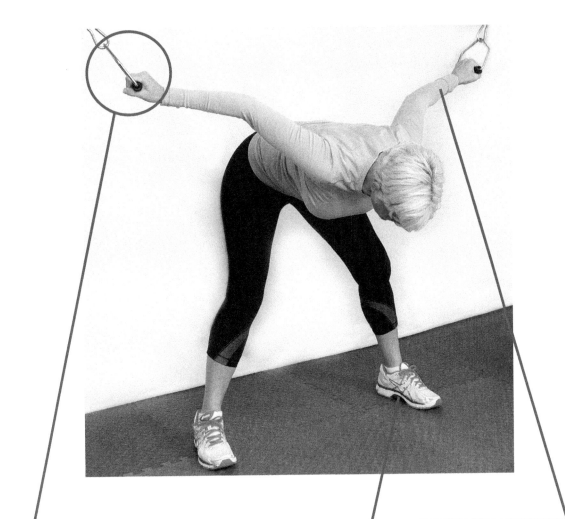

Handgrip

Use the stirrups attached to the highest cable position.

Body position

Place your feet shoulder-width apart with your knees bent and your back flat.

Arm position

Open your arms wide. Keep your elbows slightly bent.

2. Finish

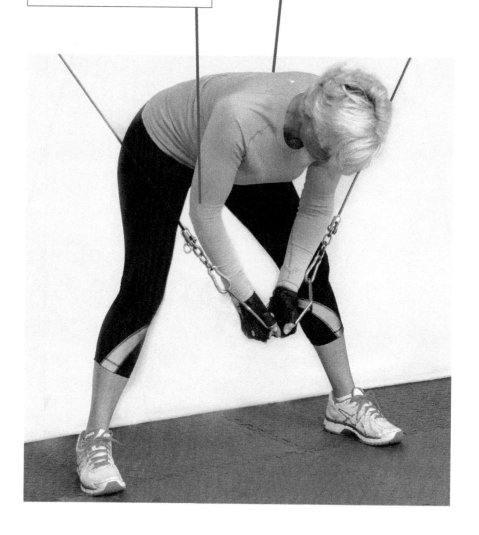

Arm position

Move your arms in an arc as if hugging a barrel. Keep your elbows slightly behind your shoulders.

Back position

Keep your back flat. *Avoid* arching.

MACHINE CHEST FLY

The machine chest fly is the least effective as the available range of motion is generally restricted. However, when using this machine arm placement is crucial: always maintain a horizontal forearm to decrease injury risk, regardless of the machine's design.

1. Start

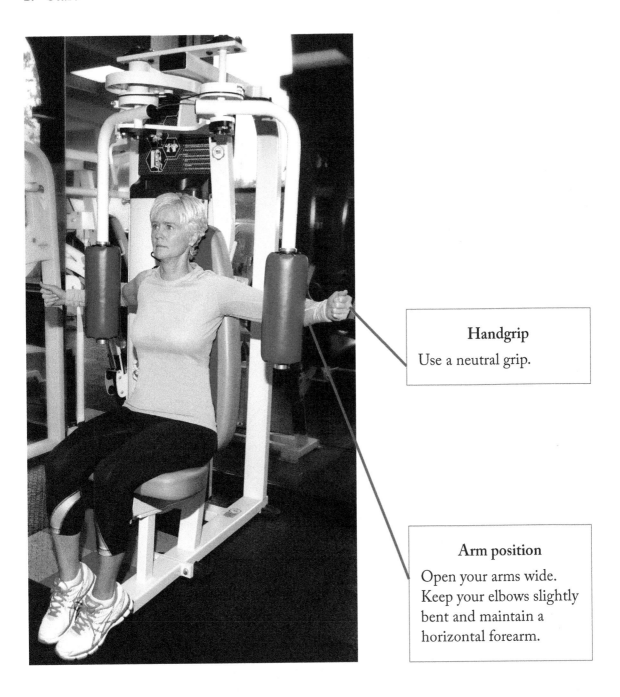

Handgrip

Use a neutral grip.

Arm position

Open your arms wide. Keep your elbows slightly bent and maintain a horizontal forearm.

2. Finish

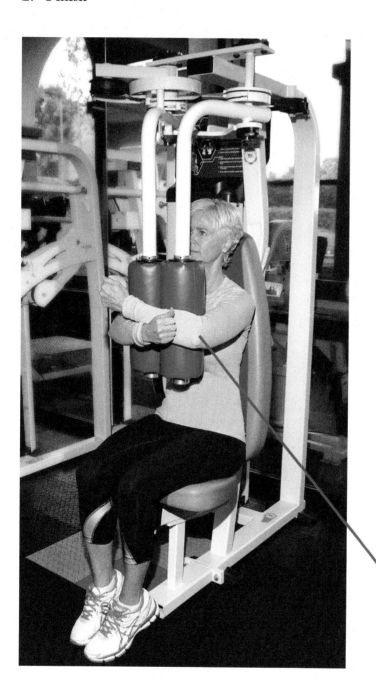

Arm position

Move your arms in an arc as if hugging a barrel. Keep your elbows slightly below your shoulders.

SECTION V

SHOULDERS

THE SHOULDER PRESS

*The shoulder press is the exercise for
enhancing the size and appearance of your shoulders.*

THE SHOULDER IS ONE OF THE most frequently injured joints in weight training, accounting for 18% of all injuries in competitive lifters.[1,2] Performing upper-body exercises improperly—most notably the bench press, as we describe in Chapter 13—can quickly lead to injury. Additionally, emphasizing larger muscle groups, such as the chest, while neglecting muscles of the back creates muscle imbalances, which predisposes the shoulder to injury.[1,3] Nevertheless, shoulder presses are beneficial for shoulder strengthening when properly executed.

You will see in this chapter how the exercise can be performed using a variety of equipment. We do not give a Master Technique for the shoulder press, as the moves presented are all equally effective.

EQUIPMENT OPTIONS

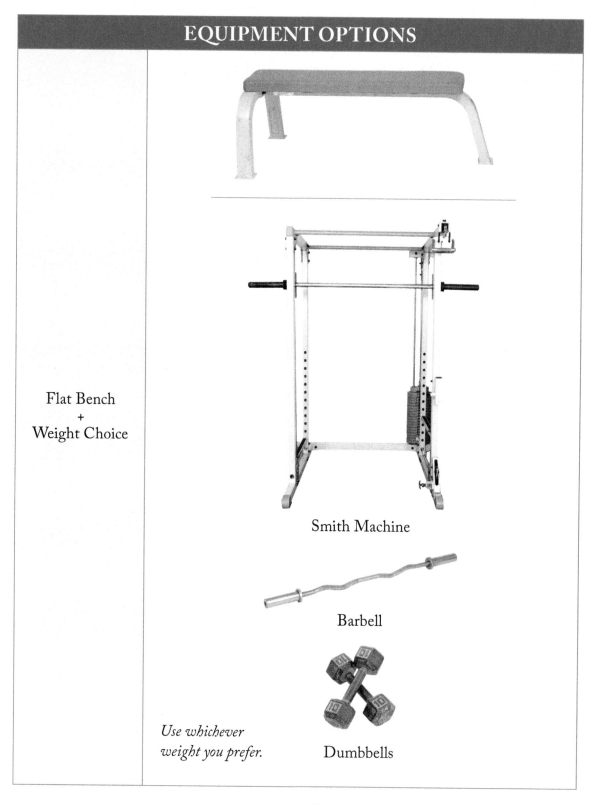

Flat Bench
+
Weight Choice

Smith Machine

Barbell

*Use whichever
weight you prefer.*

Dumbbells

Equipment options continue on the next page.

Shoulder Press
Machine

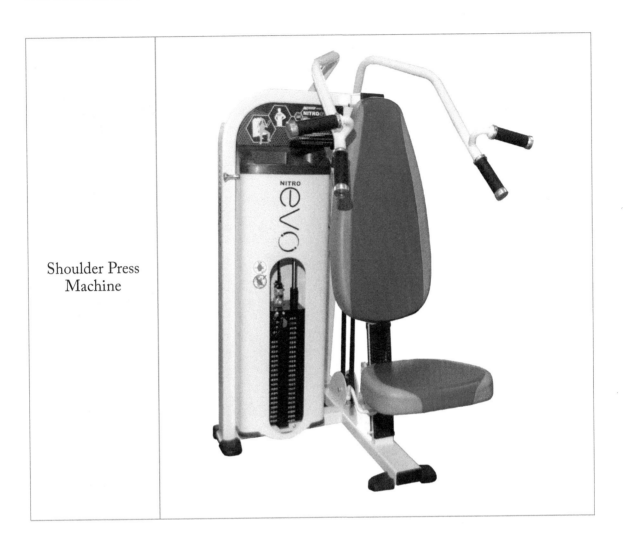

KEY POINTS FOR A SAFE
AND EFFECTIVE SHOULDER PRESS

1. Handgrip

When using dumbbells or a shoulder press machine, you often have a choice of handgrips. Choose the most comfortable.

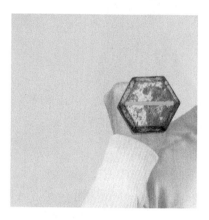

Correct

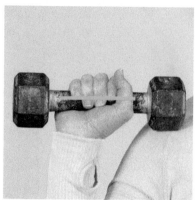

Correct

2. Weight position

Bring the weights to shoulder height to obtain a full range of motion, which is necessary to optimize muscle activity within the shoulder region.[4]

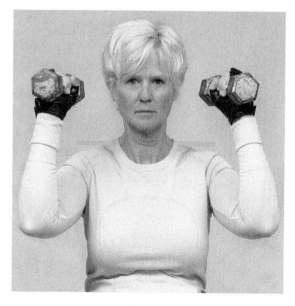

Correct

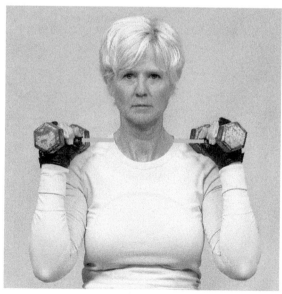

Correct (preferred)

As in the lat pulldown, the weight should *never* be positioned behind your head. Doing so can result in irreparable damage to your rotator cuff and neck.[1,5,6]

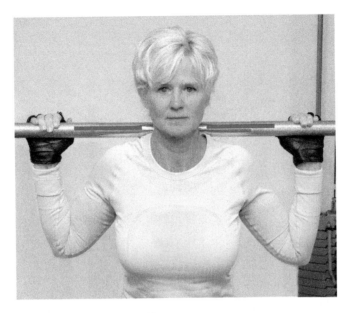

Incorrect

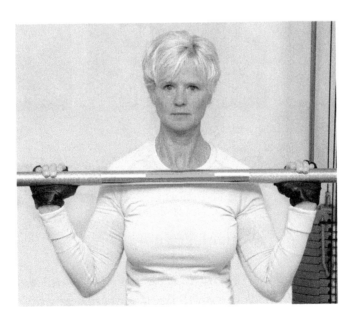

Correct

3. Arm position

Always keep your elbows in front of your shoulders to avoid shoulder injury. Any machine that forces your hands or elbows to move behind your shoulders should be avoided. If you turn your body around on such a machine, your elbows will remain in front of your shoulders.[6]

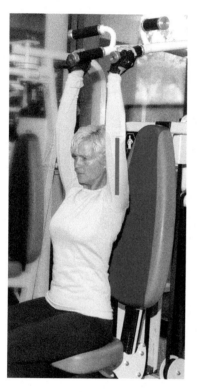
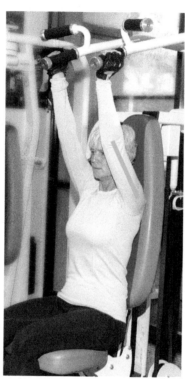
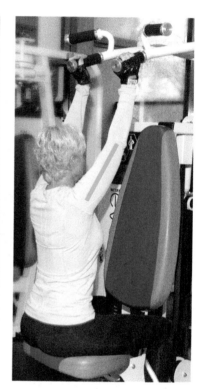

Incorrect   Correct   Correct

Weight-Training Tip

A disadvantage of any machine is that it could force you into an unnatural position. To make the predefined movements safe, some machines allow you to modify your technique (as we point out on this page and elsewhere in the book). If this is not possible, it is necessary to avoid using the machine.

SHOULDER PRESS
(USING BARBELL OR SMITH MACHINE)

The shoulder press with a barbell or Smith machine is done with the same technique. However, the Smith machine is safer—the machine stabilizes the bar.

1. **Start**

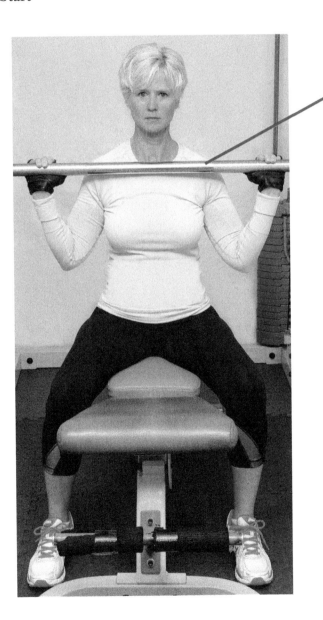

Weight position

Bring the bar to shoulder height for the full range of motion.

2. **Finish**

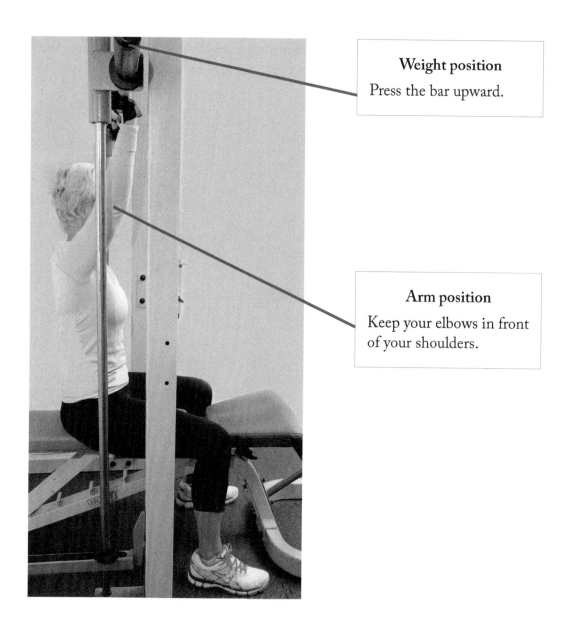

Weight position

Press the bar upward.

Arm position

Keep your elbows in front of your shoulders.

DUMBBELL SHOULDER PRESS

The main advantage of the dumbbell shoulder press is it allows you to determine if one side is stronger than the other.

1. Start

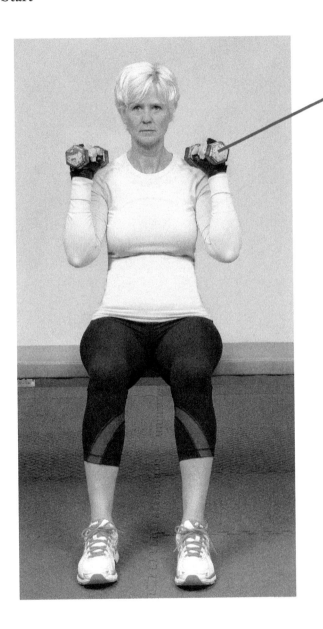

Weight position

Bring the dumbbells to shoulder height for the full range of motion.

2. Finish

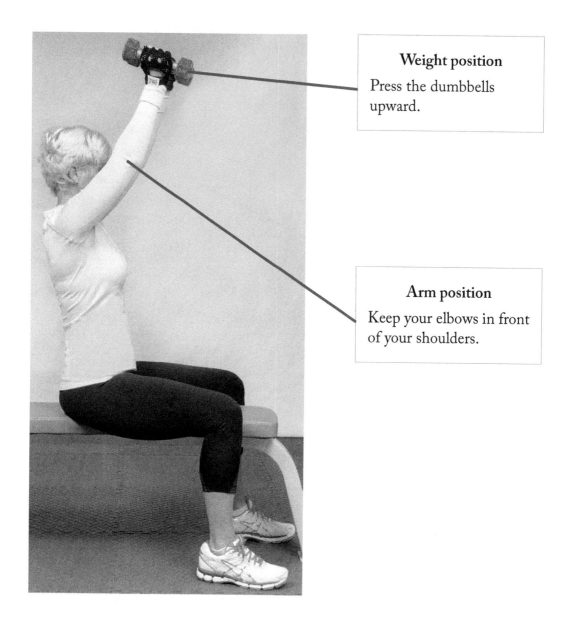

Weight position

Press the dumbbells upward.

Arm position

Keep your elbows in front of your shoulders.

MACHINE SHOULDER PRESS

Depending on the design of the machine, you may need to position yourself facing the machine (even if the manufacturer recommends facing away) to make sure your elbows remain in front of your shoulders.

1. Start

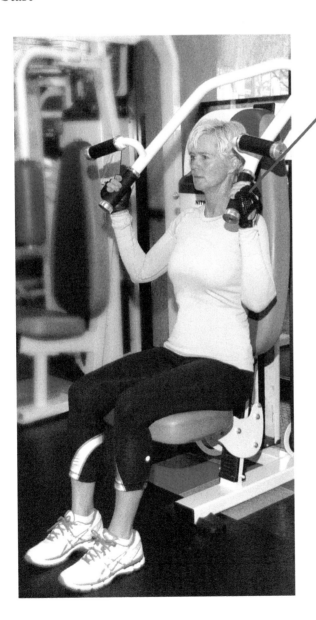

Weight position

Bring the weight to shoulder height for a full range of motion. Adjust the seat height if necessary. However, this may not be possible because of the machine's design (as shown).

2. Finish

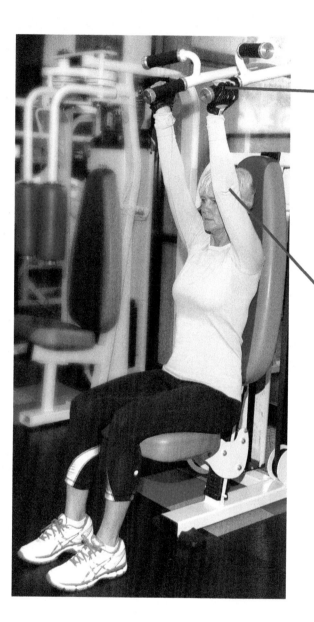

Weight position

Press the weight upward.

Arm position

Keep your elbows in front of your shoulders. Turn your body around if necessary.

THE SHOULDER RAISE

The Complete Shoulder Move, which is featured in this chapter, is one of the best shoulder exercises, and one that should be performed regularly.

GENERALLY, WEIGHT-TRAINING PROGRAMS FOR THE shoulder complex emphasize shoulder presses, which target your deltoids (the most visible muscles on top of your shoulders).[1] However, neglect of your shoulder stabilizers (particularly the rotator cuff muscles) leaves your shoulders prone to injury.[2] Therefore, shoulder raises (especially ones that target the supraspinatus—the rotator cuff muscle most frequently implicated in shoulder problems) are essential to your shoulder routine.[3]

In this chapter, we show you why the common techniques employed for shoulder raises are frequently dangerous, as well as how to perform the exercise for maximum benefit. We present Fred's favorite shoulder raise exercise, which he taught to his co-author Rachel to help Dr. Eric Grotzinger, her associate dean at Carnegie Mellon, with his frozen shoulder. Dr. Grotzinger later proclaimed, "Rachel forever changed my life and healed my frozen shoulder."

EQUIPMENT OPTIONS

Flat Bench
+
Dumbbells

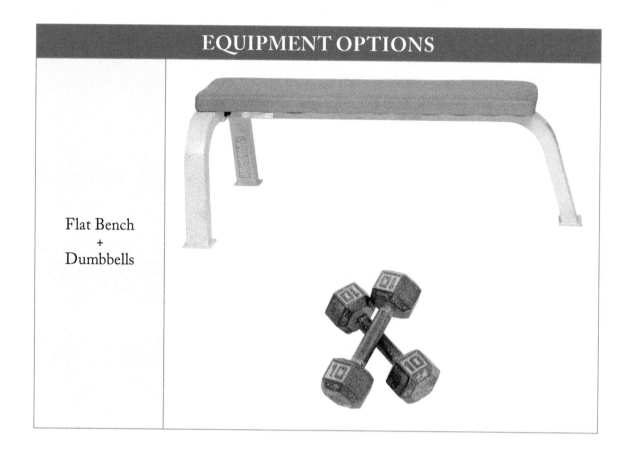

Weight-Training Tip

*Although we picture dumbbells as the equipment of choice,
any light weight (such as a pair of 16-ounce water bottles) would suffice.
In this chapter, any weight over 5 pounds would probably be too heavy.*

KEY POINTS FOR A SAFE AND EFFECTIVE SHOULDER RAISE

1. Exercises to be avoided

   Avoid lateral raises (exercises that require you to raise your arms directly to your side). Lateral raises place unnecessary stress on your shoulders and can cause shoulder impingement. *Avoid* any exercise (or machine) that requires such a movement.[4-6]

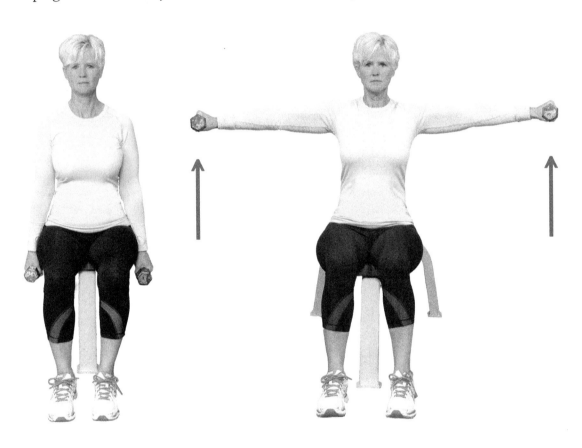

Lateral Raise (to be avoided)

2. Handgrip

Always keep your thumbs on top. Thumb-down positions are less safe (because they increase the risk of shoulder impingement) and are ineffective for strengthening the supraspinatus (because the muscle is placed at a mechanical disadvantage).[3, 6, 7]

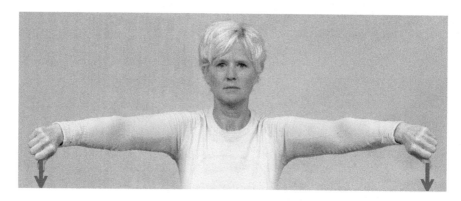

Incorrect

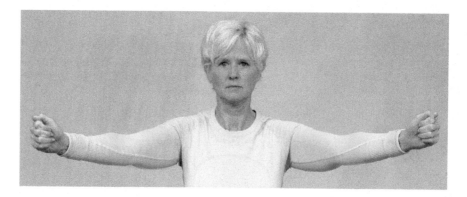

Correct

MASTER TECHNIQUE: COMPLETE SHOULDER MOVE

The *Complete Shoulder Move* is the only exercise that effectively works all the muscles of your shoulder in a single exercise with an emphasis on the supraspinatus. Perform it slowly in a controlled manner with little weight.

1. Start

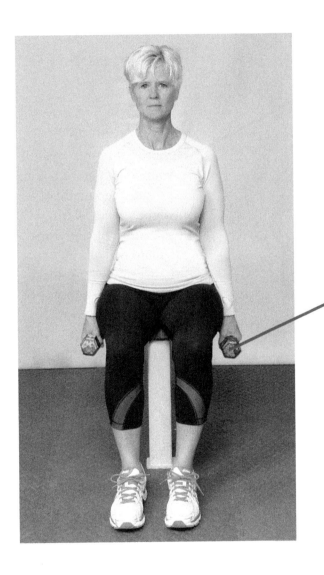

Weight position

Place the dumbbells at your side.

2. Finish (there are 4 parts)

Up

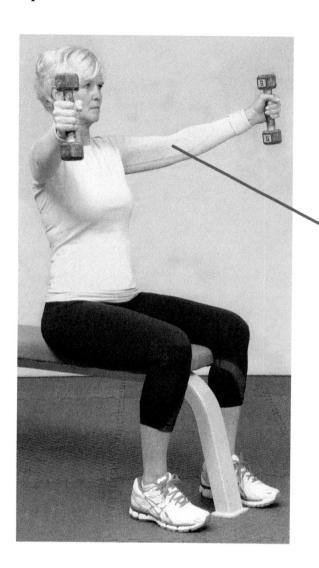

Arm position

Raise your arms *up* until your elbows are shoulder height, keeping them slightly bent. Ideally, the width of your arms should be halfway between the "together" and "wide" positions on the following pages.

Together

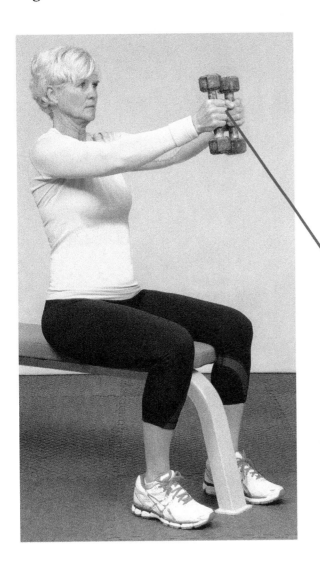

Weight position

Bring the dumbbells *together*.

Wide

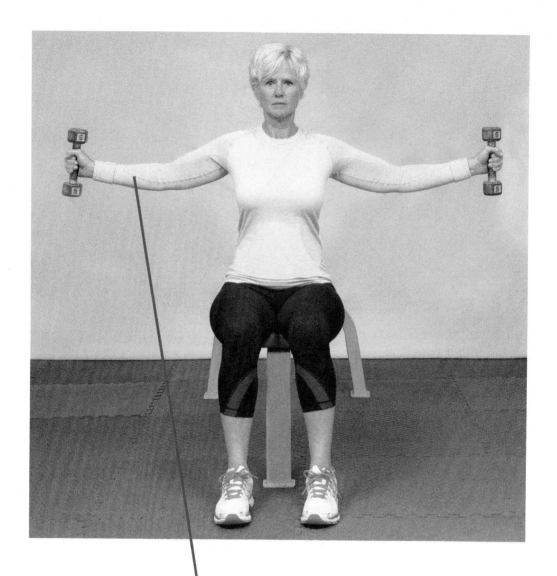

Arm position

Open your arms *wide* until they are aligned with your body.

Twist and Down

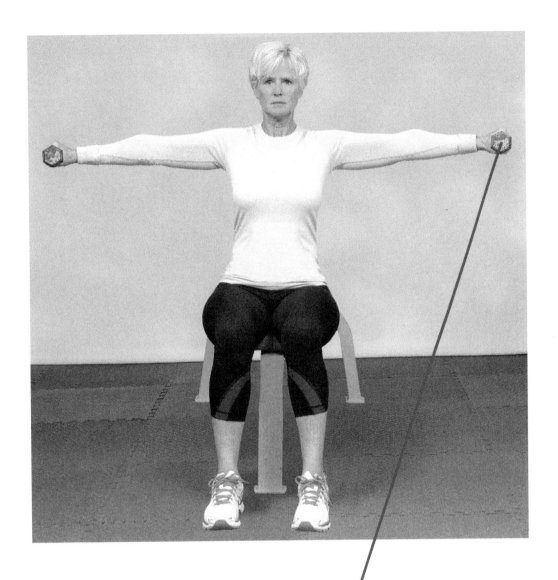

Weight position

Twist the dumbbells down and lower them slowly to your side.

SECTION VI

ARMS

THE BICEPS CURL

The biceps curl is one of the simplest, if not the simplest, upper-body exercises. Yet, people still injure themselves from improper form.

ALL FLEXING OR PULLING MOVEMENTS TOWARD your body employ your biceps (two-headed muscle in the front of your arm). If you want to achieve the most aesthetically appealing arms, biceps curls are essential. The biceps curl is a basic move, yet people tend to perform it improperly, and poor technique can lead to injury, particularly at the wrist and elbow. (Wrist and elbow injuries account for up to 9% each, together 18%, of injuries in competitive lifters.[1])

This chapter teaches you the secrets to proper biceps strengthening using the preacher bench, dumbbells, and a cable system.

EQUIPMENT OPTIONS

Preacher Bench
+
Barbell

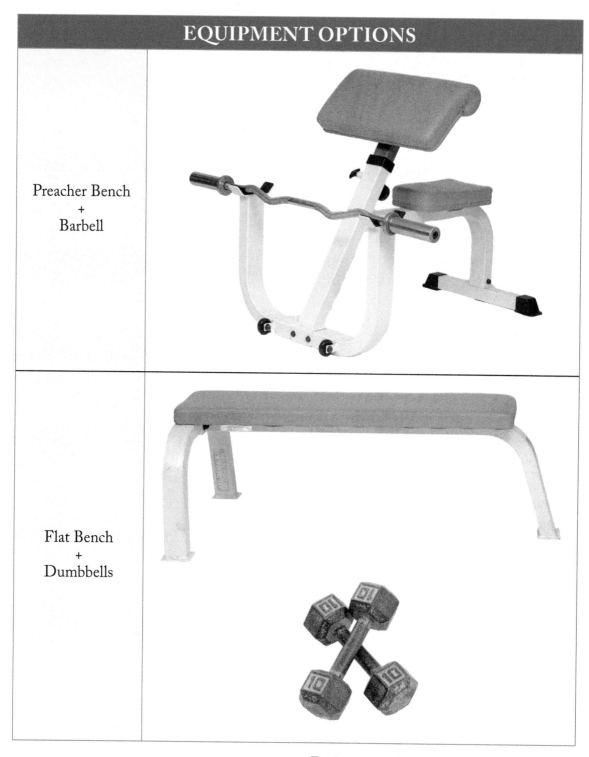

Flat Bench
+
Dumbbells

Equipment options continue on the next page.

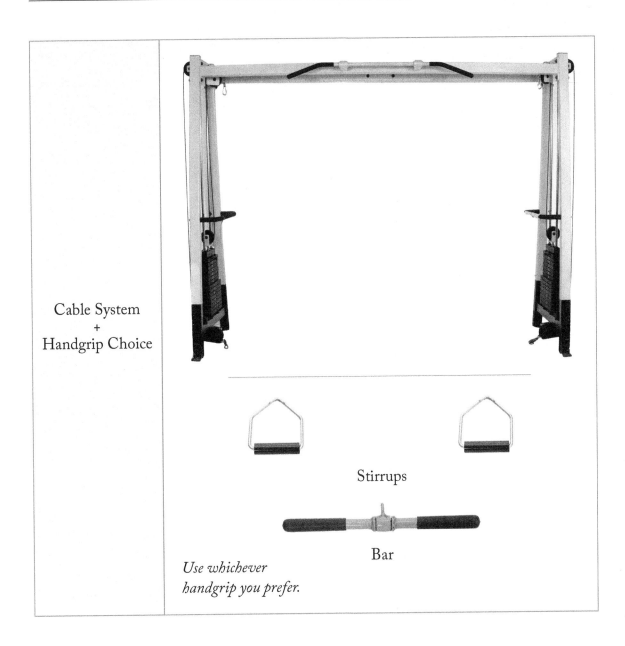

Cable System
+
Handgrip Choice

Stirrups

Bar

*Use whichever
handgrip you prefer.*

KEY POINTS FOR A SAFE AND EFFECTIVE BICEPS CURL

1. Wrist position

Keep your wrists in a natural position (*not* bent). Excessive wrist flexion (generally to compensate for the use of too much weight) overloads the muscles that bend your wrist and can precipitate elbow pain (notably medial epicondylitis, more commonly known as golfer's elbow).[2]

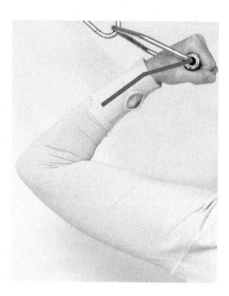 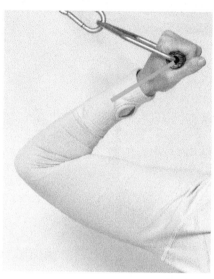

Incorrect   Correct

2. Arm position

Keep your elbows slightly bent at the full extension to eliminate stress on your elbows. Additionally, straightening your elbows (combined with the use of excessive weight) can cause tendinitis (or even rupture) of the distal biceps tendon.[3-5]

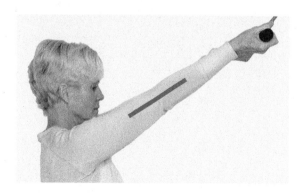 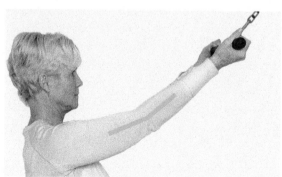

Incorrect   Correct

Avoid moving your elbows. They should pivot only. Moving your elbows increases shoulder activity and lessens biceps usage.

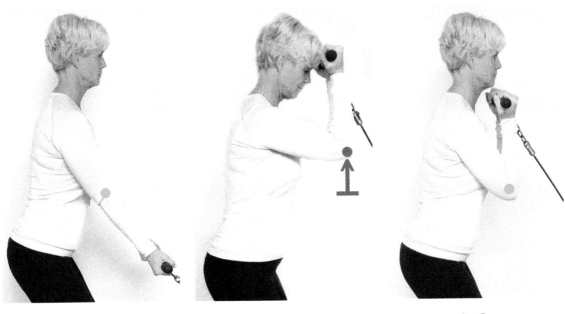

Start: Correct   Finish: Incorrect   Finish: Correct

3. **Weight position (when using dumbbells)**
   Curl the weight up and slightly outward for a full range of motion. The combination of these movements maximizes biceps activity.[6-8]

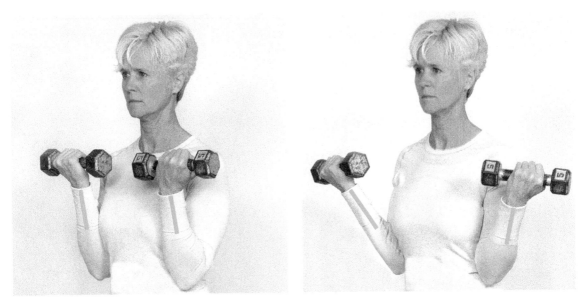

Correct   Correct (preferred)

4. **Back position**

Keep your shoulders back. Rounding your shoulders strains the muscles of your back and increases the chance of injury. This is relevant to any movement but is particularly important when your torso is forward (as for the low-cable curl with bar, as shown).

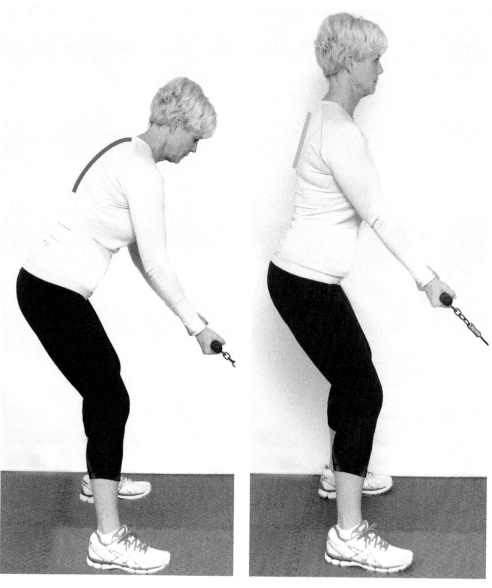

Incorrect   Correct

5. Body position

Do *not* swing your body. Swinging your body takes away from proper biceps strengthening and promotes low-back injury.

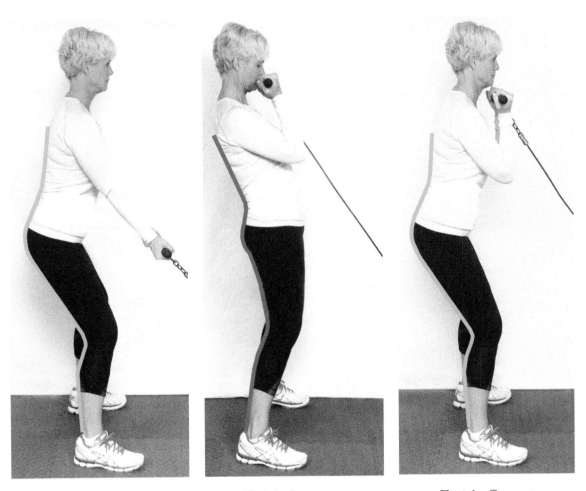

Start: Correct   Finish: Incorrect   Finish: Correct

MASTER TECHNIQUE: PREACHER CURL

The preacher curl is one of the simplest biceps moves because the bench automatically puts you in the proper position. We prefer using a barbell (as shown) because it allows for a full range of motion. Although preacher benches with an attached bar are often available and may be used, many models tend to limit the range of motion.

1. **Start**

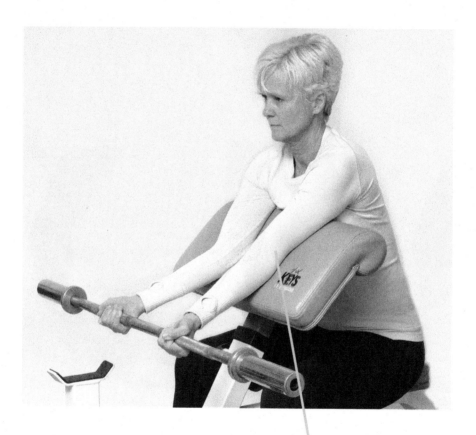

Arm position

Extend your arms. Keep your elbows slightly bent.

2. Finish

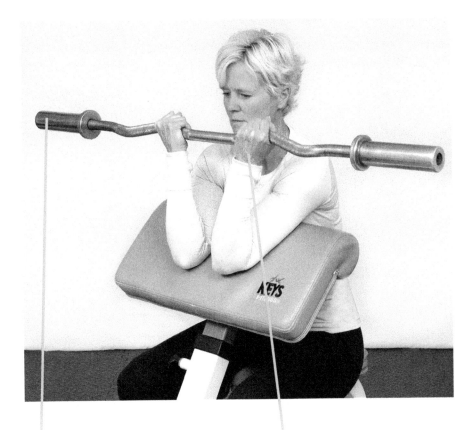

Weight position
Curl the bar upward.

Wrist position
Keep your wrists in a
natural position (*not*
bent).

Weight-Training Tip

Depending on the type of preacher curl equipment you use, you may be able to modify the position of your elbows. Keeping your elbows close (as shown above) minimizes potential strain on them and places greater emphasis on your biceps.

DUMBBELL CURL

Variation 1: Basic Dumbbell Curl

This exercise can be done seated or standing and using both arms together or one arm at a time. (We are showing this standing, but these options are all beneficial.)

1. **Start**

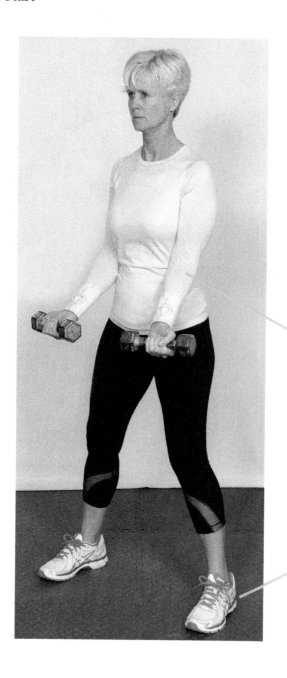

Arm position

Extend your arms. Keep your elbows slightly bent.

Body position

Place your feet shoulder-width apart with your knees bent and torso upright.

2. Finish

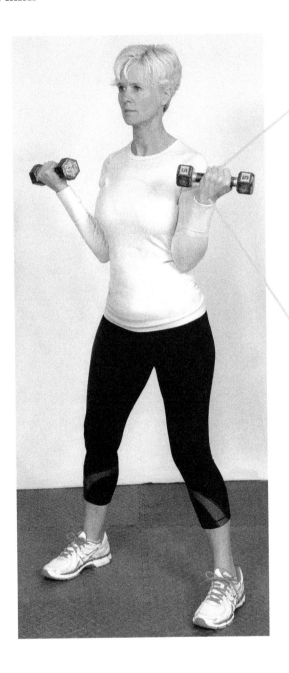

Weight position

Curl the dumbbells up and slightly outward for a full range of motion.

Wrist position

Keep your wrists in a natural position (*not* bent).

Variation 2: Concentrated Curl

The concentrated curl, as its name implies, emphasizes one arm at a time. We recommend a bench for stabilization.

1. Start

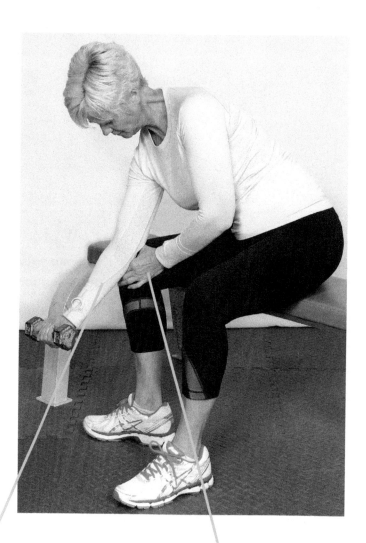

Arm position

Extend your arm. Keep your elbow slightly bent.

Wrist position

Lock your arm into a stationary position with the opposite hand to prevent slippage.

2. Finish

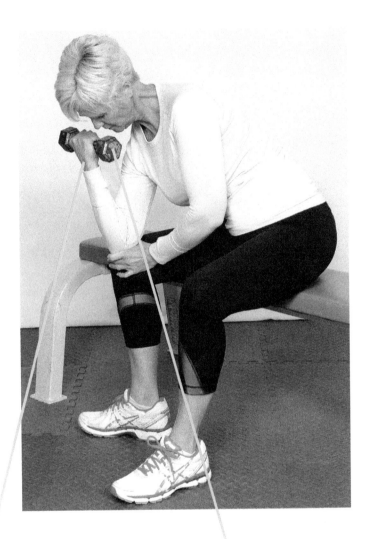

Wrist position

Keep your wrist in a natural position (*not* bent).

Weight position

Curl the dumbbell up and slightly outward for a full range of motion.

CABLE CURL

Variation 1: Low-Cable Curl with Bar

1. Start

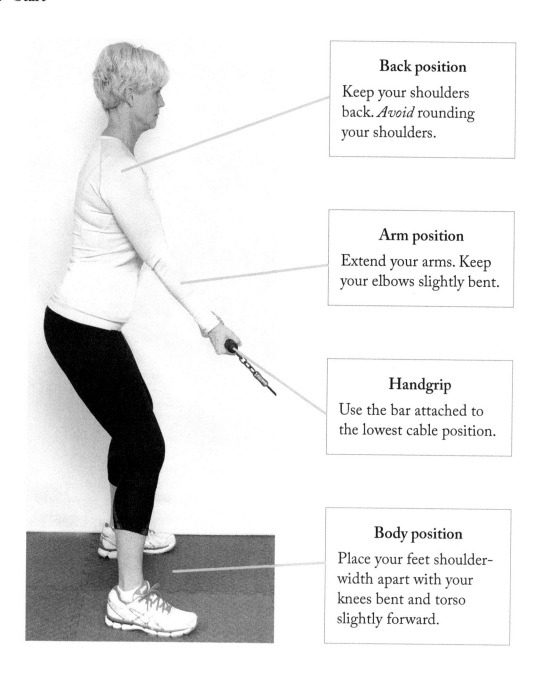

Back position

Keep your shoulders back. *Avoid* rounding your shoulders.

Arm position

Extend your arms. Keep your elbows slightly bent.

Handgrip

Use the bar attached to the lowest cable position.

Body position

Place your feet shoulder-width apart with your knees bent and torso slightly forward.

2. Finish

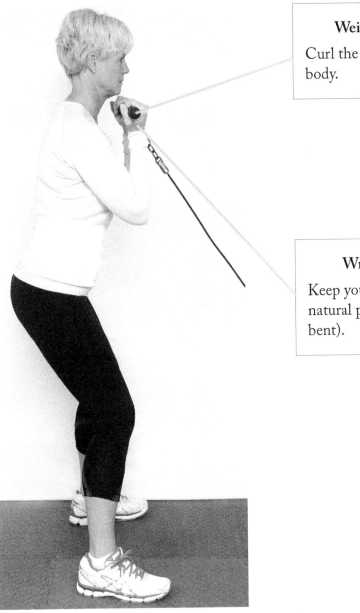

Weight position

Curl the bar toward your body.

Wrist position

Keep your wrists in a natural position (*not* bent).

Variation 2: High-Cable Curl with Bar

1. Start

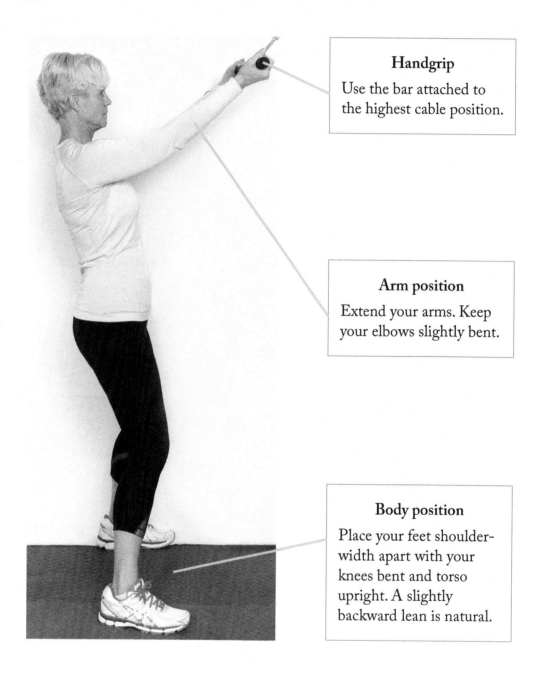

Handgrip

Use the bar attached to the highest cable position.

Arm position

Extend your arms. Keep your elbows slightly bent.

Body position

Place your feet shoulder-width apart with your knees bent and torso upright. A slightly backward lean is natural.

2. Finish

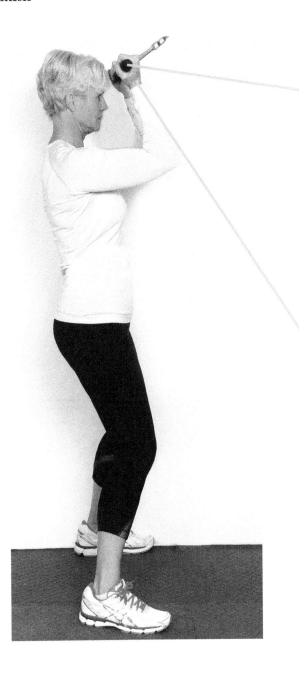

Weight position

Curl the bar to your forehead.

Wrist position

Keep your wrists in a natural position (*not* bent).

Variation 3: High-Cable Curl with Stirrups

For a more sculptured biceps, perform this move in two stages: one set curling to your forehead (Stage 1), and a second set curling to the back of your head (Stage 2).

1. **Start**

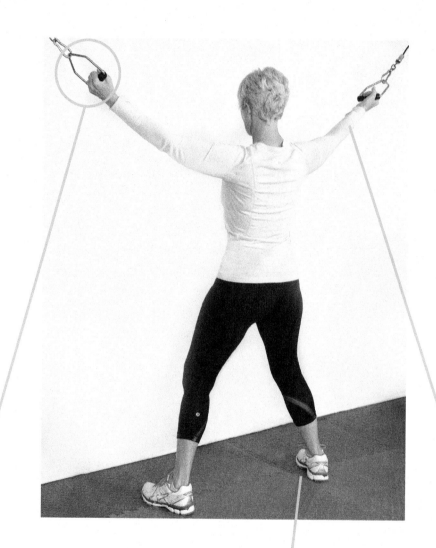

Handgrip

Use the stirrups attached to the highest cable position.

Body position

Place your feet shoulder-width apart with your knees bent and torso upright.

Arm position

Extend your arms. Keep your elbows slightly bent.

2. Finish

Stage 1

Wrist position

Keep your wrists in a natural position (*not* bent).

Weight position

Curl the stirrups to your temples.

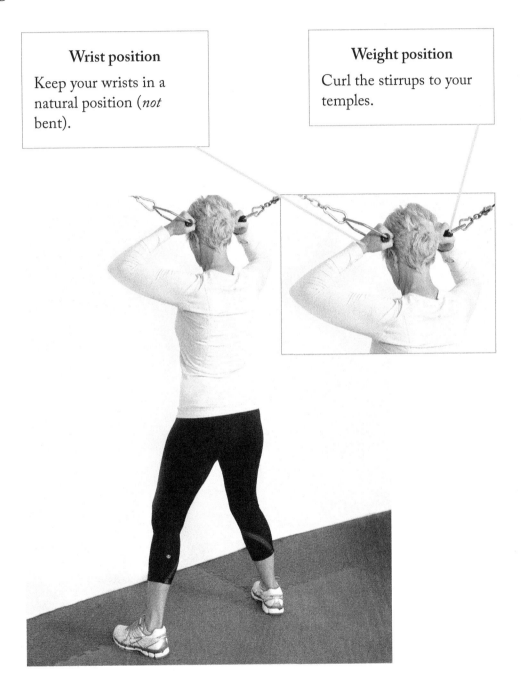

Stage 2

> **Wrist position**
>
> Keep your wrists in a natural position (*not* bent).

> **Weight position**
>
> Curl the stirrups to the back of your head.

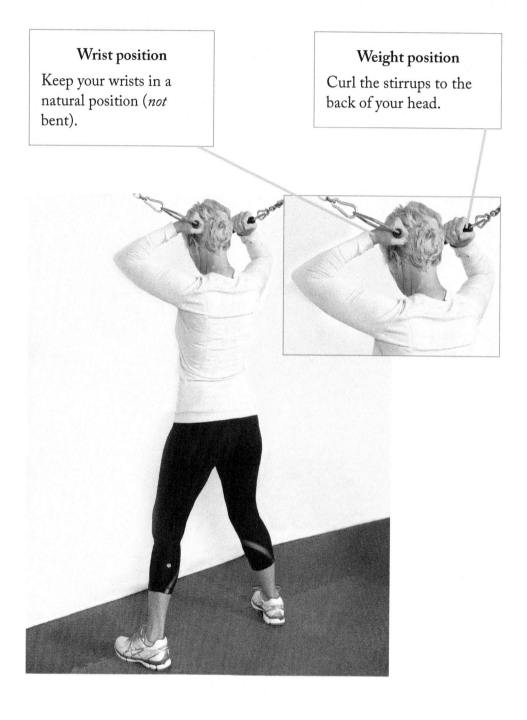

THE TRICEPS EXTENSION

*Do you have a second wave or loose underdeveloped
muscle in your upper arm? Do you want more attractive arms?
If the answer to either of these questions is "yes," then you need
to strengthen your triceps, the largest muscle in your upper arm.*

WHENEVER YOU MAKE ANY EXTENDING OR pushing move, you use your triceps (three-headed muscle in the back of your upper arm). Even though you may commonly perform such movements, the triceps are generally not isolated, which explains why your arms may be underdeveloped.

In this chapter, we show you the secrets to optimizing your triceps workout, using a cable system, dumbbells, and a barbell. You will soon discover that proper hand placement is essential to avoid injury and achieve the best results.

EQUIPMENT OPTIONS

Cable System
+
Handgrip Choice

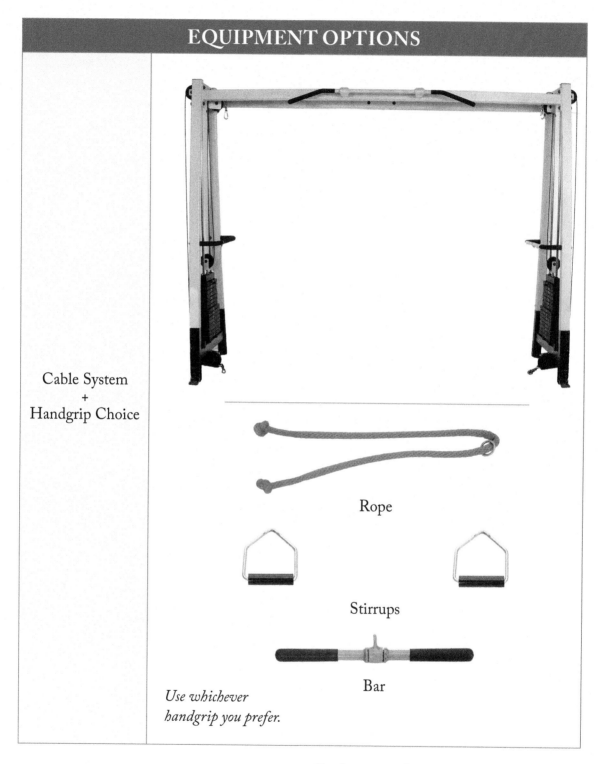

Rope

Stirrups

Bar

*Use whichever
handgrip you prefer.*

Equipment options continue on the next page.

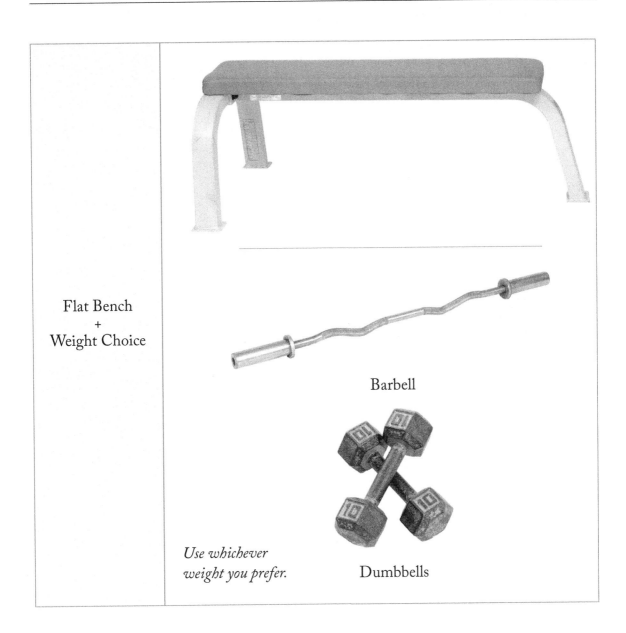

Flat Bench
+
Weight Choice

Barbell

*Use whichever
weight you prefer.*

Dumbbells

KEY POINTS FOR A SAFE AND EFFECTIVE TRICEPS EXTENSION

1. Handgrip

Place your hands in the position that keeps your elbows close to your body. This helps target your triceps, lessen shoulder activity, and protect your elbows from injury. Your palms should be facing you whether you are using a barbell or a bar.

Using a Barbell

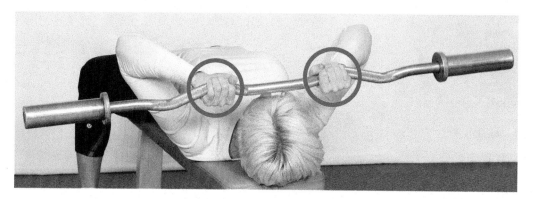

Incorrect

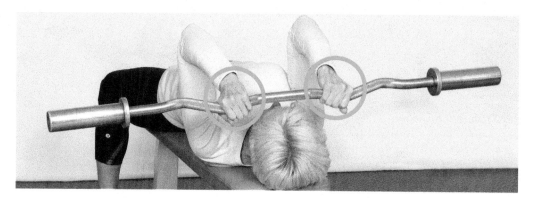

Correct

Using a Bar

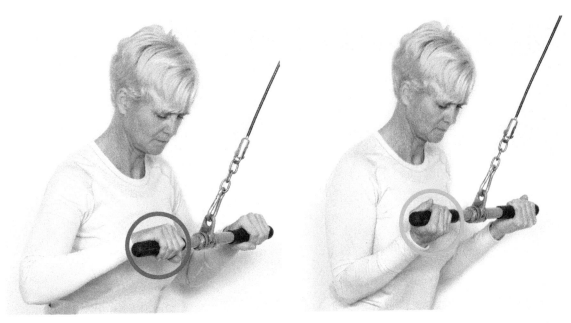

Incorrect   Correct

2. Arm position

Avoid moving your elbows up and down. They should pivot only.

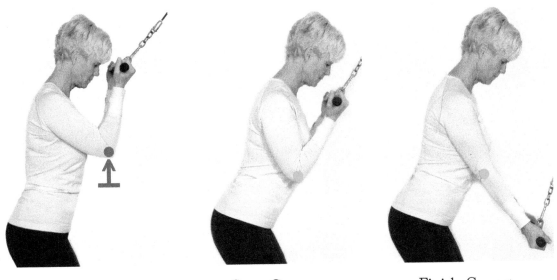

Start: Incorrect   Start: Correct   Finish: Correct

Avoid flaring your elbows. Flaring your elbows increases shoulder activity, lessens triceps usage, and places unnecessary stress on your elbows.

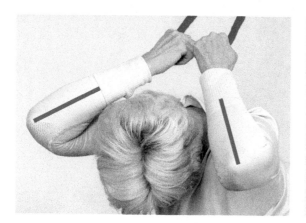 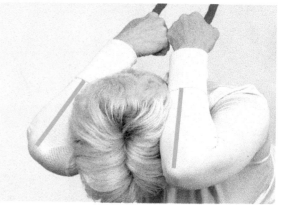

Incorrect   Correct

Extend your arms completely to achieve a full range of motion. Unlike biceps exercises where extending your elbows can cause injury, full elbow extension during triceps exercises is necessary and non-stressful to your elbows. This is because the type of muscle contraction is different for the two types of exercises—eccentric during biceps curls and concentric during triceps extensions—which influences the load at your elbows.

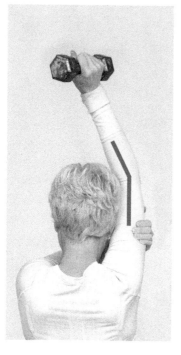 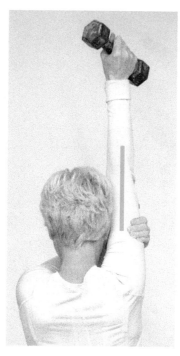

Correct   Correct (preferred)

3. Back position

Keep your shoulders back. Rounding your shoulders lessens triceps activity and strains the muscles of your back. This is relevant to any movement but is particularly important when your torso is forward (as for the rope pushdown, pictured below).

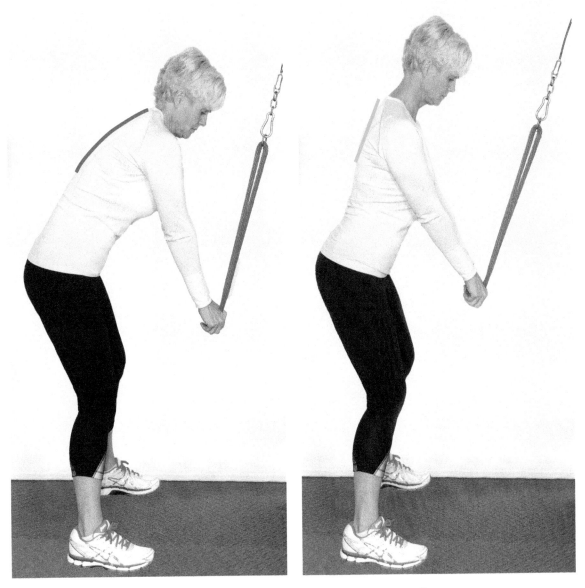

Incorrect   Correct

Keep your back flat. Rounding your back increases the chance of injury, particularly to your low back. This is only relevant to movements in which your torso is parallel to the ground (as for the dumbbell kickback, as shown).

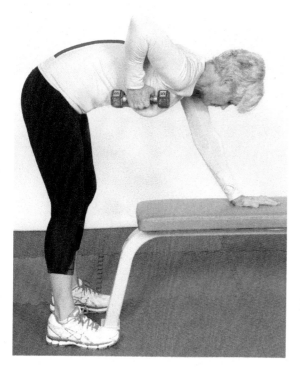
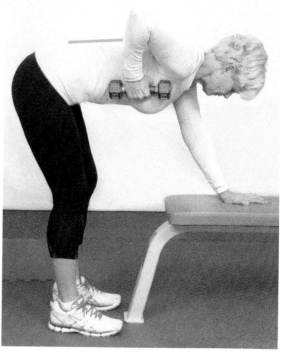

Incorrect   Correct

Weight-Training Tip

*The position of your torso during different exercises
will vary (as we show repeatedly throughout this book).
Always remember: your torso position should maximize the benefit
of the exercise but, at the same time, minimize your risk of back injury.*

MASTER TECHNIQUE: CABLE TRICEPS EXTENSION (USING ROPE)

A rope is the most effective method for working your triceps. Ropes that are found at most gyms are thick, short, and difficult to grip, like the common triceps rope, pictured below on the left. We recommend a thinner and longer rope, like the Stellabotte Triceps Enhancer Rope, pictured below on the right.

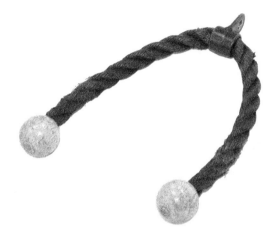

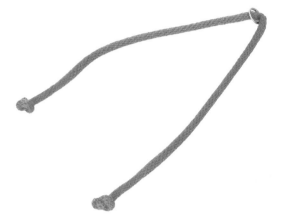

Common Triceps Rope   Stellabotte Triceps Enhancer Rope

The Stellabotte Triceps Enhancer Rope

The thinner type of rope is not found at gyms, but you may find out more about the Stellabotte Triceps Enhancer Rope at www.WeightTrainingWOI.com/products and learn how to obtain it. Alternatively, make your own following the steps below.

1. Purchase a piece of rope you find comfortable to grip (check out your local hardware stores). The rope should be approximately the length of your arm (from shoulder to wrist), or 2 feet, but since the rope must be folded, you need to buy 4 feet.
2. Purchase a metal ring. This will allow you to attach the rope to the machine.
3. Thread the rope through the metal ring then tie off the ends.

Variation 1: Rope Pushdown

1. Start

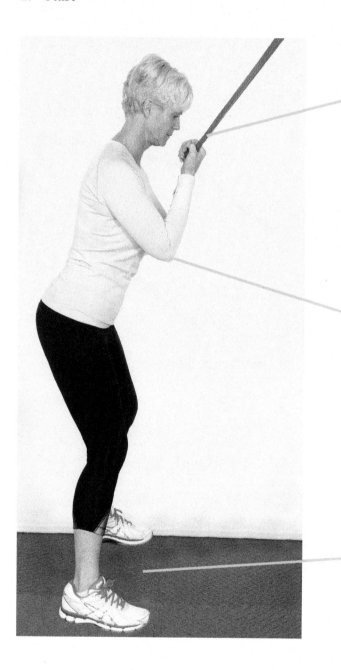

Handgrip

Use the rope attached to the highest cable position. Begin with the rope near your face.

Arm position

Keep your elbows close to your body.

Body position

Place your feet shoulder-width apart with your knees bent and torso slightly forward.

2. Finish

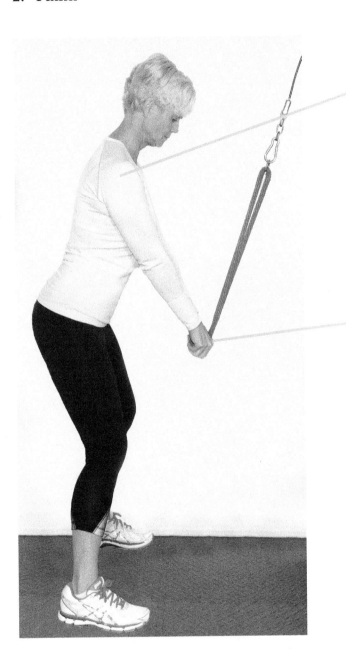

Back position

Keep your shoulders back. *Avoid* rounding your shoulders.

Arm position

Extend your arms completely down to achieve a full range of motion.

Variation 2: Rope Overhead Extension

1. Start

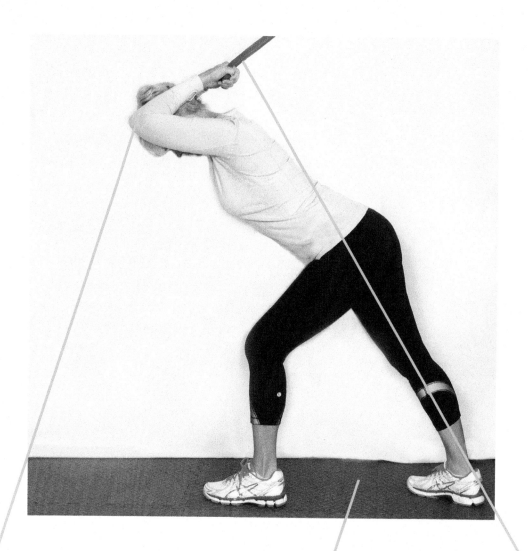

Arm position

Keep your elbows close to your head.

Body position

Place your feet shoulder-width apart (or in a staggered stance, as shown) with your knees bent and torso forward.

Handgrip

Use the rope attached to the highest cable position. Bring it back behind your head for a full range of motion.

2. Finish

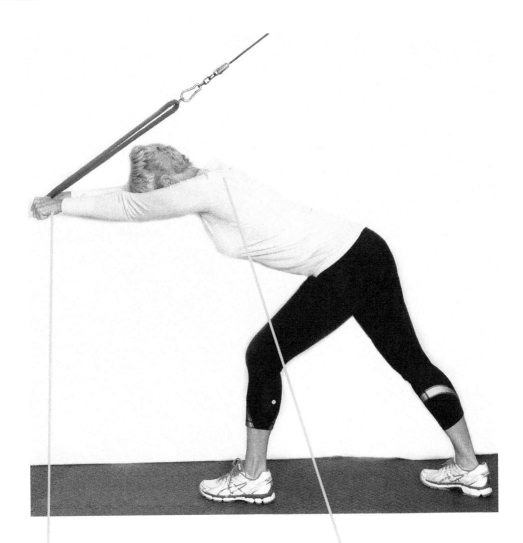

Arm position

Extend your arms completely forward to achieve a full range of motion.

Back position

Keep your shoulders back. *Avoid* rounding your shoulders.

CABLE TRICEPS EXTENSION
(USING BAR OR STIRRUP)

Variation 1: Bar Pushdown

1. Start

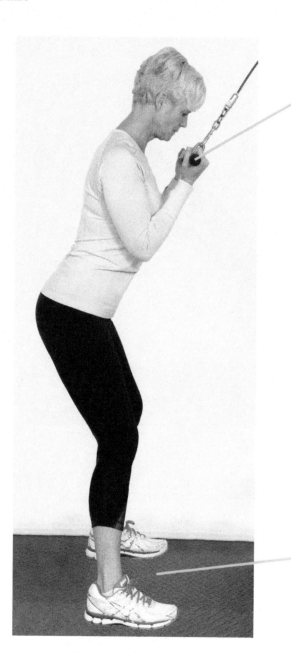

Handgrip

Use the bar attached to the highest cable position. Place your hands palms up to prevent your elbows from flaring.

Body position

Place your feet shoulder-width apart with your knees bent and torso slightly forward.

2. Finish

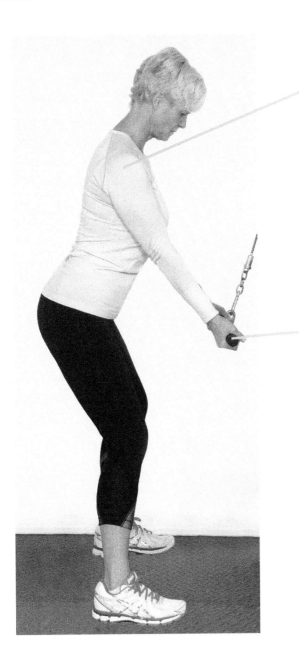

Back position

Keep your shoulders back. *Avoid* rounding your shoulders.

Arm position

Extend your arms completely down to achieve a full range of motion.

Variation 2: Stirrup Kickback

1. Start

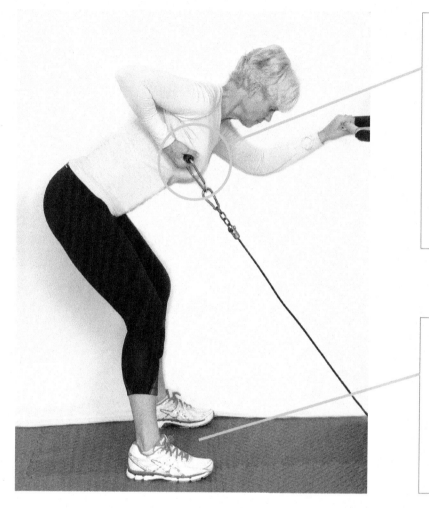

Handgrip

Use the stirrup attached to the lowest cable position, beginning with it close to your underarm. Place your hand palm up to prevent your elbow from flaring.

Body position

Place your feet shoulder-width apart with your knees bent and torso forward. Keep your shoulders back.

2. Finish

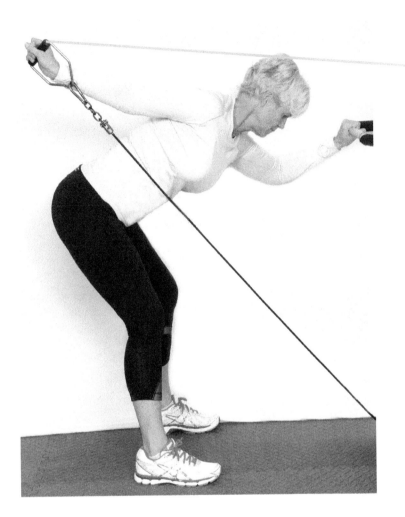

Arm position

Extend your arm up and back.

Weight-Training Tip

Throughout the book, we tell you to bend your knees and place your feet shoulder-width apart. In case you are wondering why, it is to stabilize your body. A stable stance is known as an athletic position. The position of your torso will vary with the exercise.

DUMBBELL TRICEPS EXTENSION

Variation 1: Dumbbell Kickback

This move is a variation of the stirrup version (see page 208). We recommend a bench for stabilization.

1. Start

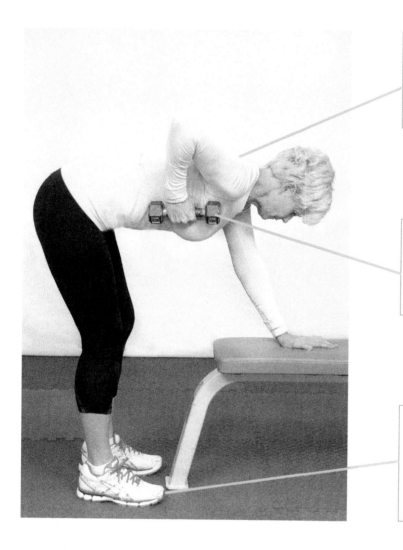

Back position

Keep your back flat. *Avoid* arching.

Weight position

Begin with the dumbbell close to your underarm.

Body position

Place your feet shoulder-width apart with your knees bent.

2. Finish

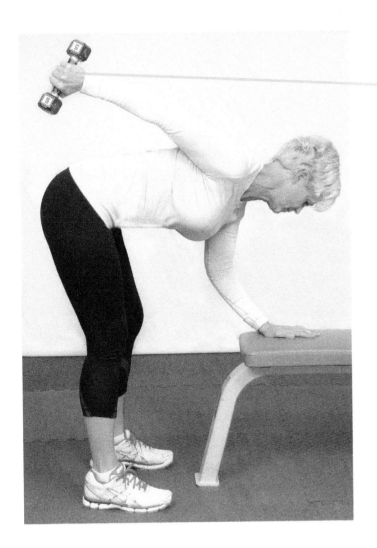

Arm position

Extend your arm up and back.

Variation 2: Seated Dumbbell Triceps Extension

This move is most effective when using one arm (as shown), as opposed to two arms simultaneously.

1. Start

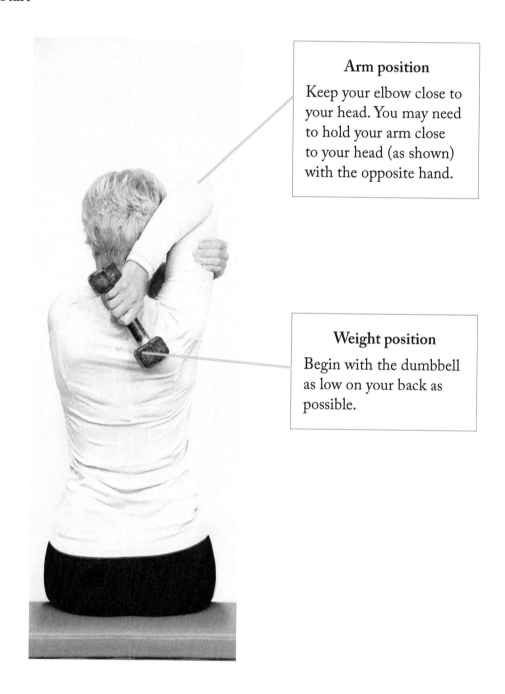

Arm position

Keep your elbow close to your head. You may need to hold your arm close to your head (as shown) with the opposite hand.

Weight position

Begin with the dumbbell as low on your back as possible.

2. Finish

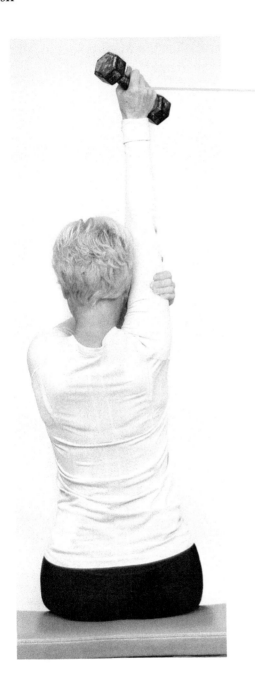

Arm position

Extend your arm up completely for a full range of motion.

Variation 3: Supine Dumbbell Triceps Extension

Some refer to this move as a "skull crusher." However, if the weight does touch your head, you are not getting the full range of motion. Rather, the weights should fall to the side of your head. This allows for a greater range of motion and is more effective.

1. **Start**

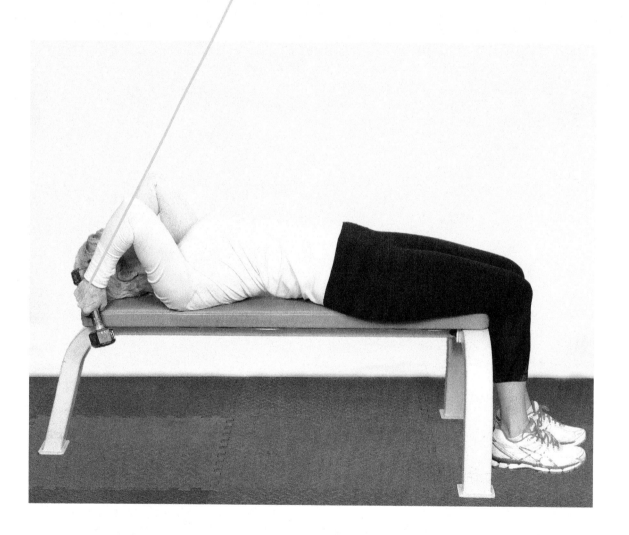

Weight position

Bring the dumbbells down to the side of your head.

2. Finish

Arm position

Extend your arms up completely for a full range of motion.

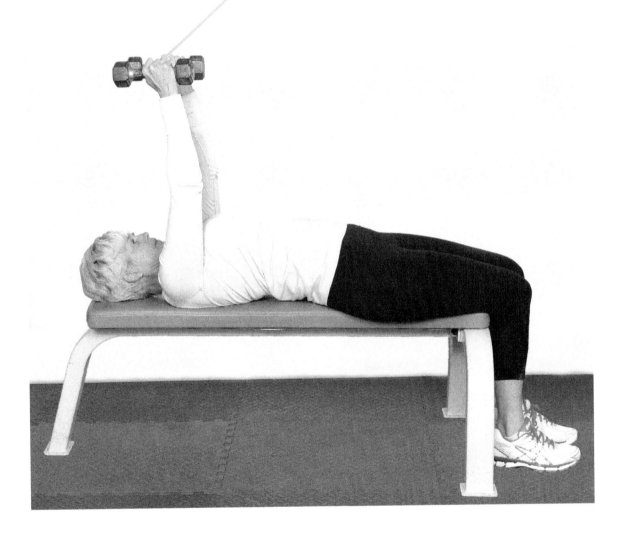

SUPINE BARBELL TRICEPS EXTENSION

This move is a variation of the dumbbell version (see page 214).

1. Start

Handgrip

Place your hands palm down to prevent your elbows from flaring.

Weight position

Begin with the bar behind your head.

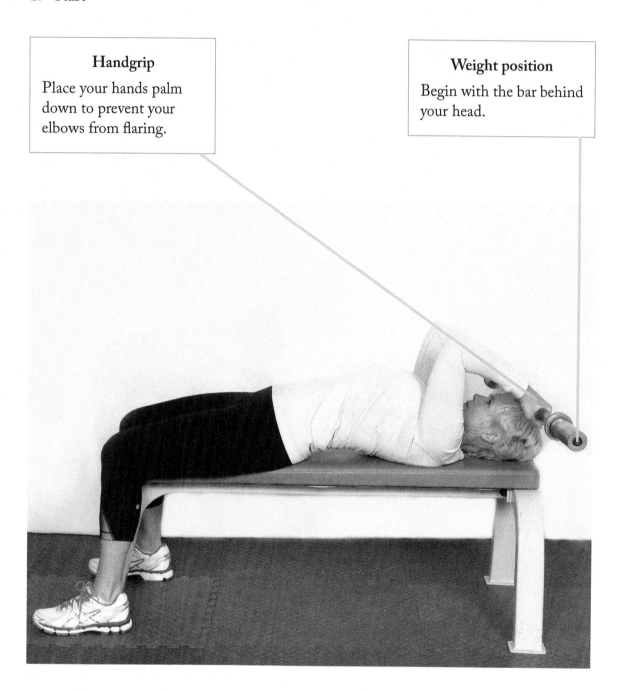

2. Finish

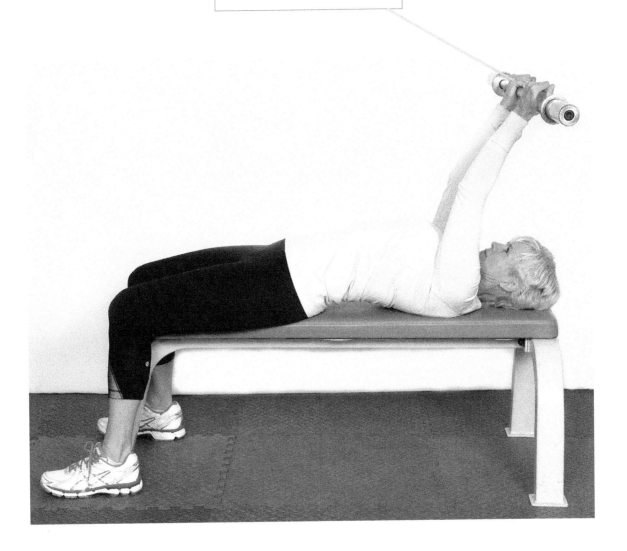

Arm position

Extend your arms up completely for a full range of motion.

SECTION VII

CORE

THE CRUNCH

Why do people do crunches? They do them for appearance.
However, the secret to attractive and appealing abdominals
is most importantly diet—in other words, mouth control!

YOU HAVE DOUBTLESS HEARD OF THE "core"—the fitness industry buzzword that refers to the 29 muscles surrounding your lumbar spine. This includes the abdominals, glutes, and back muscles.[1]

A comprehensive core routine should emphasize all the muscles surrounding the spine. Your leg and back workouts, therefore, are essential for a strong and stable core. Research indicates that squats can produce greater back muscle activation than standard "core exercises" and comparable abdominal activation.[2]

Despite the evidence, crunches and sit-ups are typically the most frequently performed exercises for the core (specifically the abdominal region). Considering that daily activities require little "curling-the-torso" strength, sit-ups and crunches should be a low priority in your workouts, while the core exercises in "The Leg Raise" (Chapter 20) and "The Plank" (Chapter 21) should generally be a higher priority.

This chapter outlines the differences between the crunch and the sit-up, and why you should always avoid the latter.

EQUIPMENT OPTIONS

Stability Ball	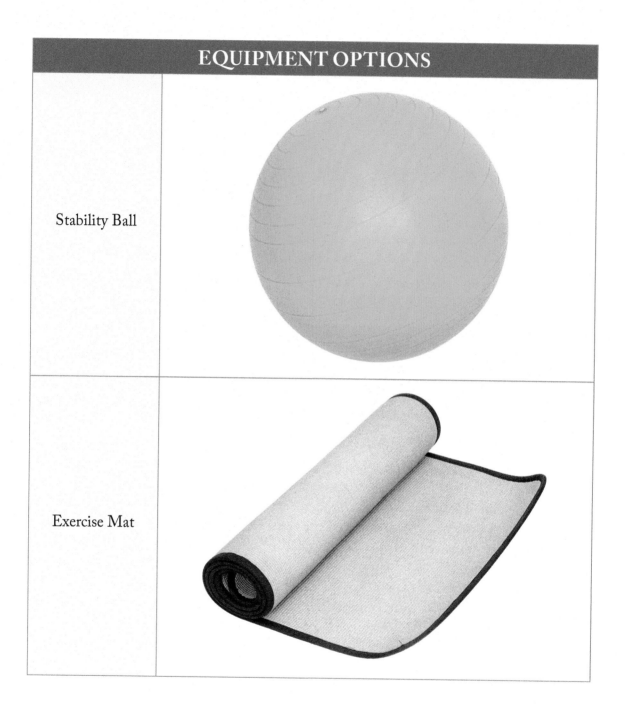
Exercise Mat	

KEY POINTS FOR A SAFE AND EFFECTIVE CRUNCH

1. **Exercises to be avoided**

    Avoid sit-ups (as shown below). Sit-ups require torso flexion until your elbows touch your knees and result in higher spinal disc compression and lower abdominal muscle activity compared with crunches.[3,4] Crunches, which are shown later in this chapter, require torso flexion until your shoulders are just off the supporting surface and are definitely the safer choice.

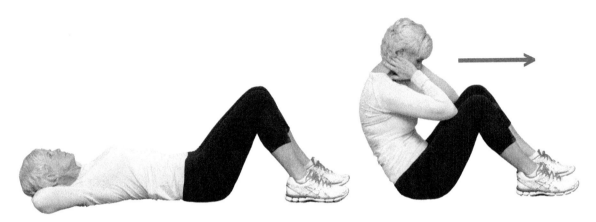

Sit-up (to be avoided)

2. **Head position**

    Keep your head in a natural position (aligned with your upper back) to avoid neck strain. Specifically, do *not* bend your neck forward.[3]

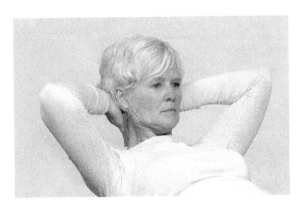

Incorrect

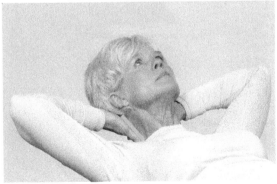

Correct

3. Arm position

All of the following arm positions are acceptable. Choose the position that enables you to get the most repetitions while maintaining proper form.

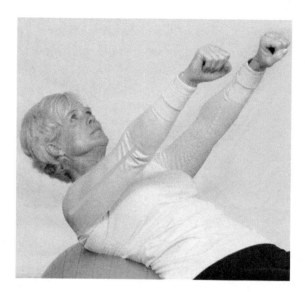

Easiest

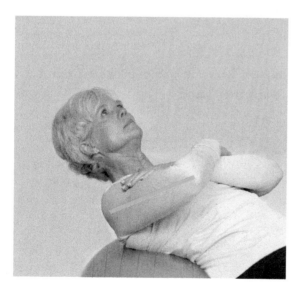

Harder

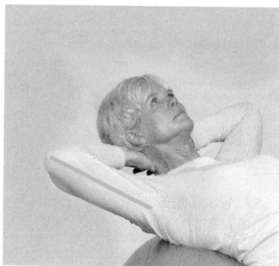

Hardest

4. Back position (for the floor crunch)

Always keep your low back supported. It should not arch. Placing your hands under your low back while keeping one leg extended will help. Alternate which leg is bent between sets.[5]

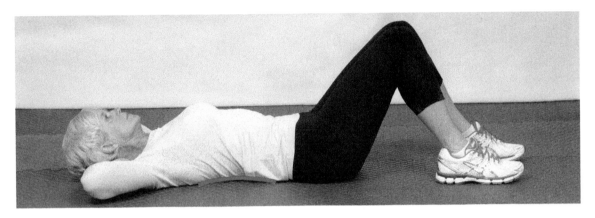

Incorrect

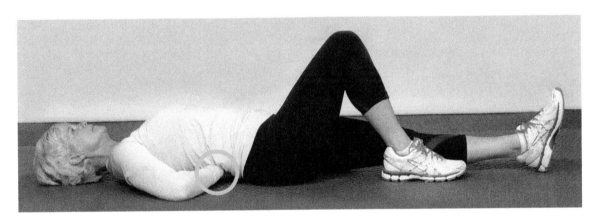

Correct

5. Foot position

Never hook your feet under any object. Hooking your feet increases activation of your hip flexors (front hip muscles), which tends to cause your low back to arch, precipitating low back pain.[3]

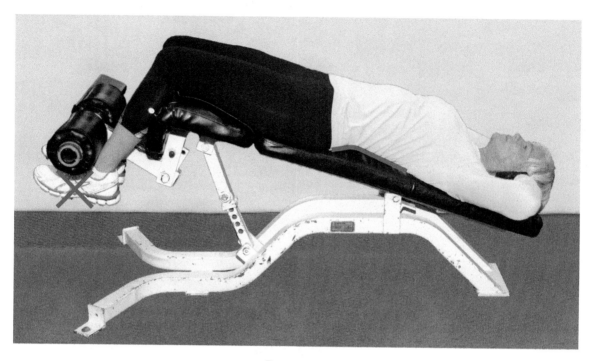

Incorrect

Weight-Training Tip

If hooking your feet is required for stabilization (as in the picture above, using a decline bench), you should not perform that exercise. On a flat surface (illustrated in the following crunch exercises), it is not necessary to hook your feet; however, if you feel the need to do so, either (a) you are executing the move incorrectly, such as doing a sit-up, which we advise against in this chapter or (b) you lack core strength (stabilization), which suggests that you need to spend more time on your overall core routine.

MASTER TECHNIQUE: STABILITY BALL CRUNCH

The crunch has been touted as one of the most effective abdominal exercises. Do one thing to ensure its effectiveness: perform the crunch using a stability ball.[6,7] The ball allows for a fuller range of motion, making the move more beneficial. Please note: The smaller the ball, the harder the move.

1. Start

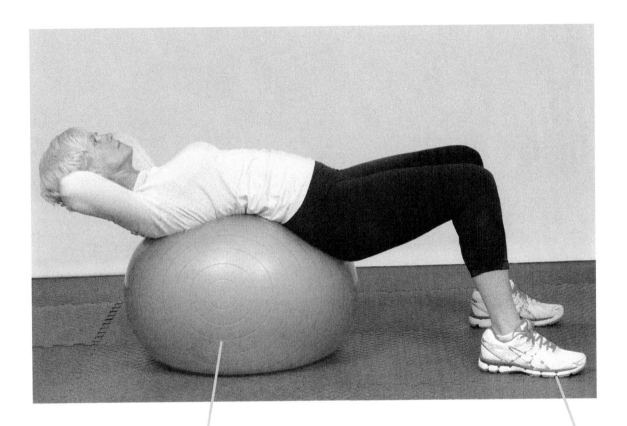

Ball position

Position the ball to support your low back.

Foot position

Place your feet against something stable for increased support if needed (such as a wall, not shown).

2. Finish

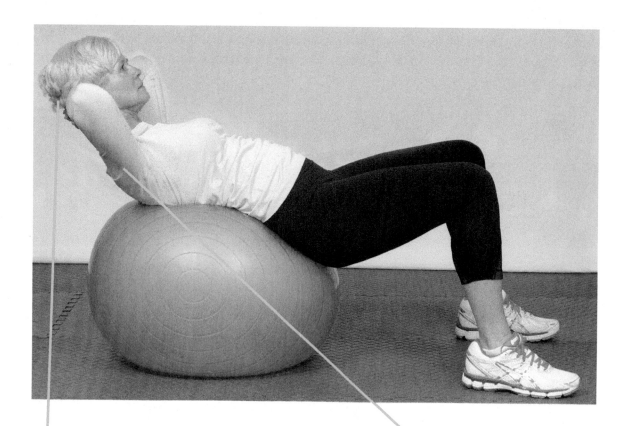

Head position

Keep your head in a
natural position. Do *not*
bend your neck forward.

Back position

Raise your torso until
your shoulders are just
off the ball.

FLOOR CRUNCH

The floor crunch works the abdominals, but it tends to be less effective than the ball version.[2] For back safety, be sure your low back remains supported.

1. Start

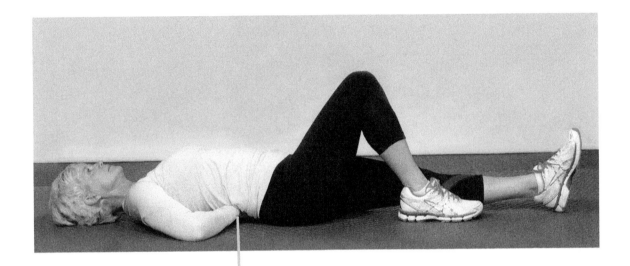

Back position

Keep your low back supported. Use your hands.

2. Finish

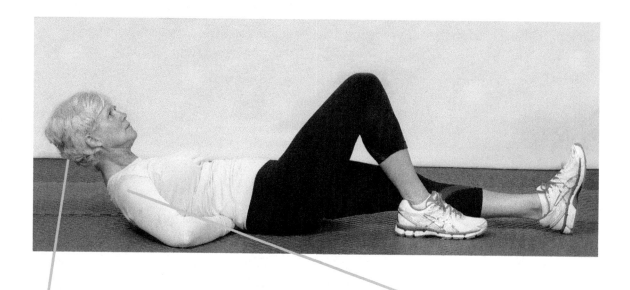

Head position

Keep your head in a natural position. Do *not* bend your neck forward.

Back position

Raise your torso until your shoulders are just off the ground.

THE LEG RAISE

The leg raise is generally the preferred exercise to tone the abdominals. It targets the lower region, which requires the most attention. However, if done improperly, the low back will be strained.

THE LEG RAISE IS CONSIDERED A nontraditional abdominal exercise. While performing the leg raise (unlike the traditional crunch), the torso does not flex; rather, the movement occurs primarily at the hip.[1] This in turn activates the muscles surrounding the lumbar region—the core—to maintain a neutral spine. Some experts refer to such movements as "lumbar stabilization" exercises.[2,3]

Without adequate core strength, leg raises will quickly increase the likelihood of back troubles.[1,4] Leg raises increase hip flexor activity, which results in pelvis rotation and hence pain, if the core muscles are not properly activated to stabilize the pelvis.

In this chapter, we instruct you on proper leg raise technique—making it possible to improve your core strength without causing injury.

EQUIPMENT OPTIONS

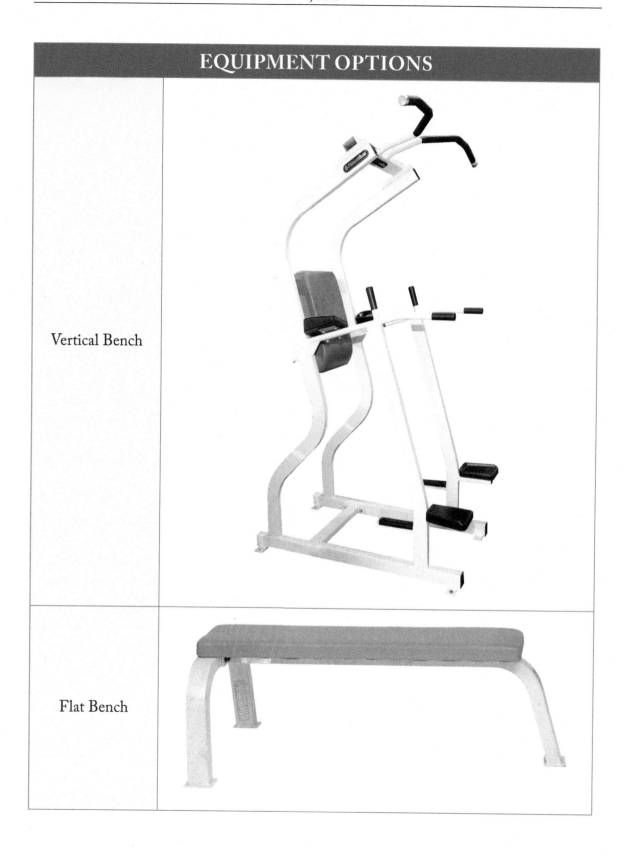

Vertical Bench

Flat Bench

KEY POINTS FOR A SAFE AND EFFECTIVE LEG RAISE

1. **Exercises to be avoided**

   Avoid straight leg raises, which tend to place improper pressure in your abdominal region. Also, *avoid* lowering your legs with your knees straight, since this requires high core muscle activation to stabilize your pelvis.[3] Without adequate core strength, your low back will arch, which in turn promotes injury.

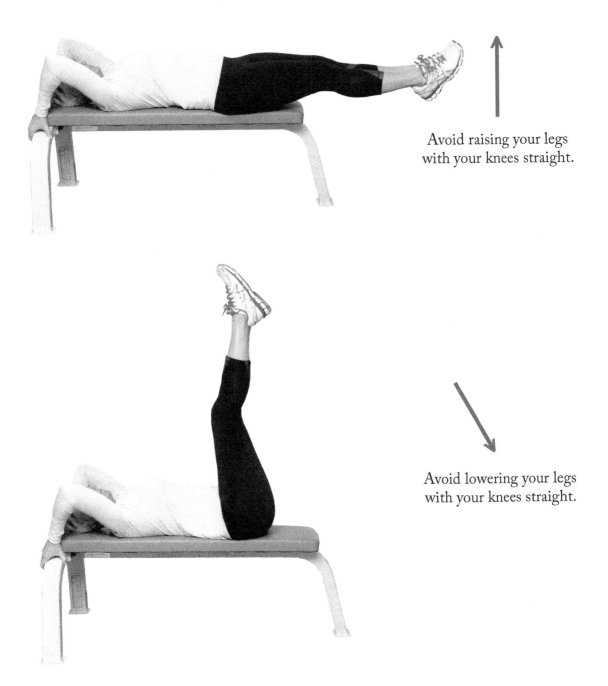

Avoid raising your legs with your knees straight.

Avoid lowering your legs with your knees straight.

MASTER TECHNIQUE:
LEG RAISE WITH VERTICAL BENCH

The leg raise from a vertical position is almost impossible to do incorrectly. We advise bending your knees at the finish (as shown) for back safety.

1. Start

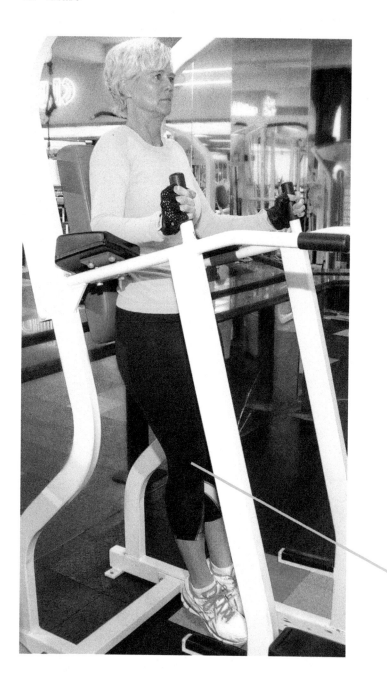

Leg position

Begin with your legs in a vertical position. Keep your knees slightly bent to protect your low back.

2. Finish

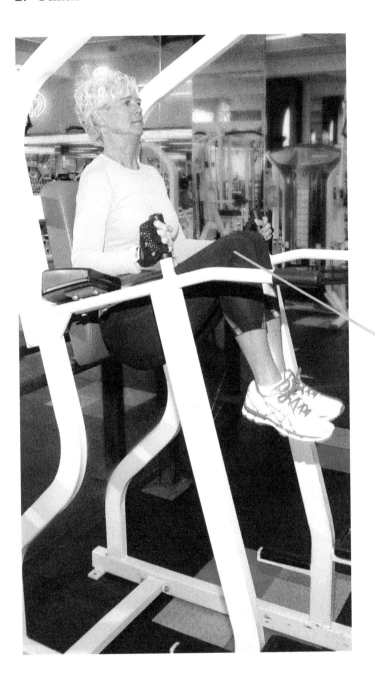

Leg position

Bring your knees up as high as possible.

LEG RAISE WITH FLAT BENCH

This exercise requires simultaneous bending at your torso and knees, which helps stabilize your low back.

1. Start

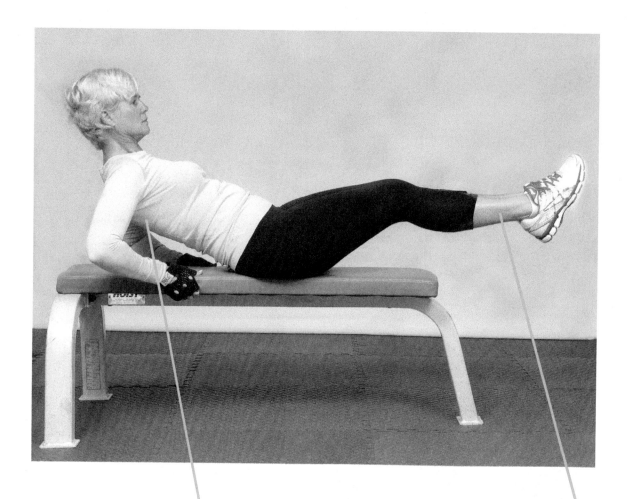

Back position

Lean your torso back.

Leg position

Extend your legs so they are horizontal to the floor. Maintain a slight bend in your knees to protect your low back.

2. Finish

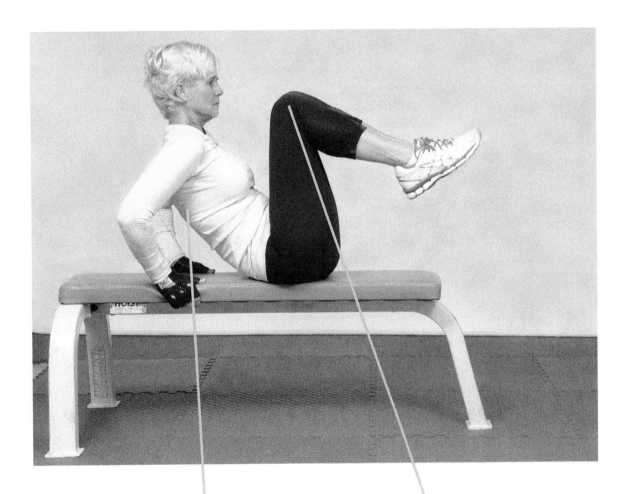

Back position
Bring your torso forward.

Leg position
Bring your knees toward your chest as far as possible.

21

THE PLANK

The plank is one of the safest core exercises, yet people tend to get bored with it. The push-up, a plank variation, is much more effective.

ACTIVITIES THAT REQUIRE LITTLE OR NO movement of the torso and minimize forces at the lumbar spine are generally the safest core exercises. One such move, the plank, requires holding a prone (face-down) position until you can no longer do so. It may be used to improve core muscle endurance—the ability to maintain a force for a period of time.[1,2]

However, boredom does tend to be an issue with this exercise, which tends to lead to improper form. As an alternative, in this chapter we propose related movements (such as push-ups), which in our opinion are more effective.

EQUIPMENT OPTIONS

Stability Ball	
Exercise Mat	
Elevated Surface	

KEY POINTS FOR A SAFE AND EFFECTIVE PLANK

1. Hand position (for the push-up)

Any of the hand positions pictured below (either close together, shoulder-width, or wide apart) are acceptable. Hand position has little influence on chest activation (that is, on the pectoralis major muscle), but narrower positions emphasize your triceps and shoulder-width (or wider) positions target your serratus anterior (muscle along the side of your ribs that facilitates proper shoulder function and alignment of your shoulder blades).[3]

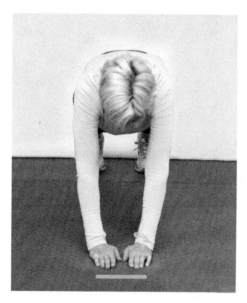

Correct (close together)

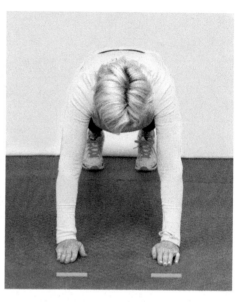

Correct (shoulder width)

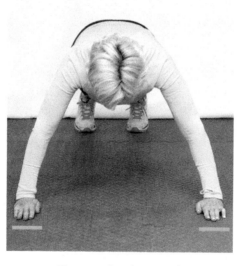

Correct (wide apart)

2. Back position

Avoid arching your low back excessively—it should maintain its natural position (slightly curved). Arching your low back excessively (generally to compensate for inadequate core stability) can injure it.

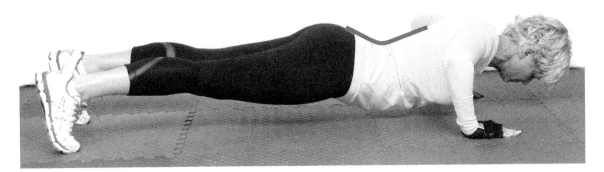

Incorrect

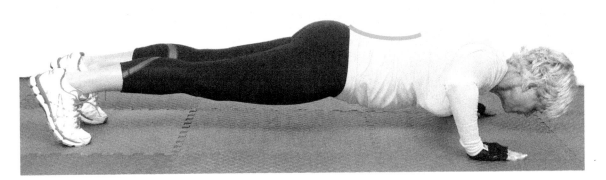

Correct

MASTER TECHNIQUE: PUSH-UP

The push-up is a variation of the plank with the added advantage of improving upper-body strength. Although it is commonly recommended for upper-body development, it does also target your entire core.[4,5]

Variation 1: Floor Push-up

1. **Start**

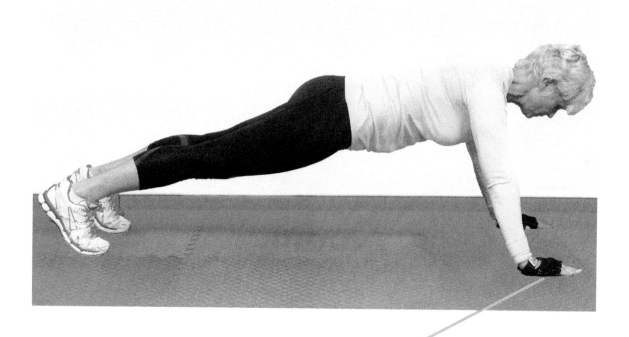

Hand position

Place your hands close together, shoulder-width, or wide apart.

2. Finish

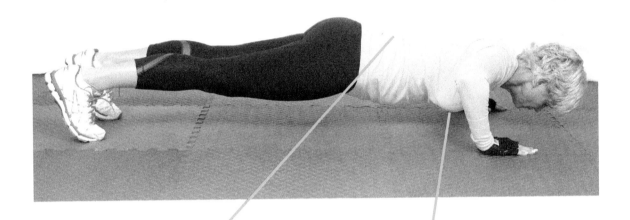

Back position

Keep your low back in its natural position (slightly curved).

Body position

Lower your body as far as possible without touching the floor.

Variation 2: Push-up on an Elevated Surface

If the floor push-up is too challenging, there's an alternative—use an elevated surface. While knee push-ups are more commonly recommended, push-ups using an elevated surface are more effective in activating your core.

1. **Start**

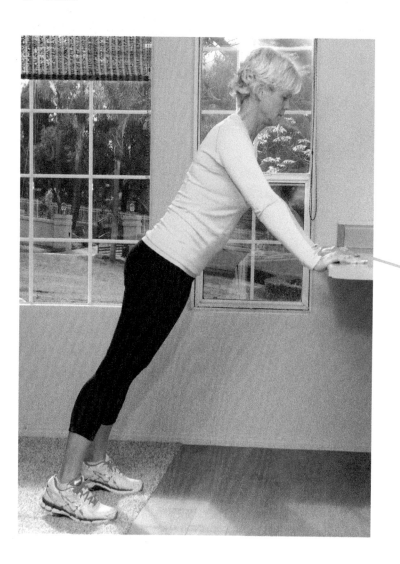

Hand position

Place your hands close together, shoulder-width, or wide apart.

2. Finish

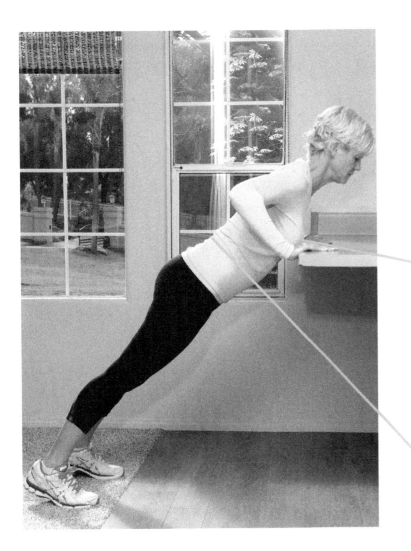

Body position

Lower your body as far as possible without touching the elevated surface.

Back position

Keep your low back in its natural position (slightly curved).

PLANK

The ability to hold a plank position is a measure of core stabilization and endurance.[1] However, the secret to enhancing core endurance is not to attempt long duration holds, but rather to do more repetitions of shorter duration (for example, 10 seconds per rep).[6]

1. Start and Finish

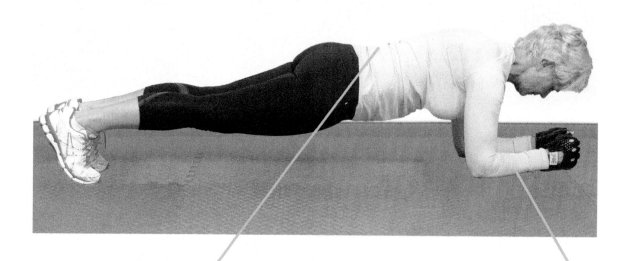

Back position

Keep your low back in its natural position (slightly curved).

Arm position

Rest on your forearms for the most stability.

STABILITY BALL PLANK CURL

The stability ball plank curl is one of the most effective exercises for your core.[8]

1. Start

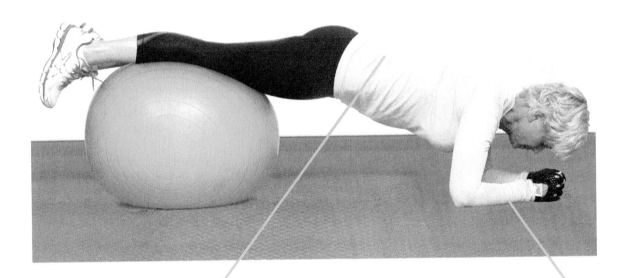

Back position
Keep your low back in its natural position (slightly curved).

Arm position
Rest on your forearms for the most stability.

2. Finish

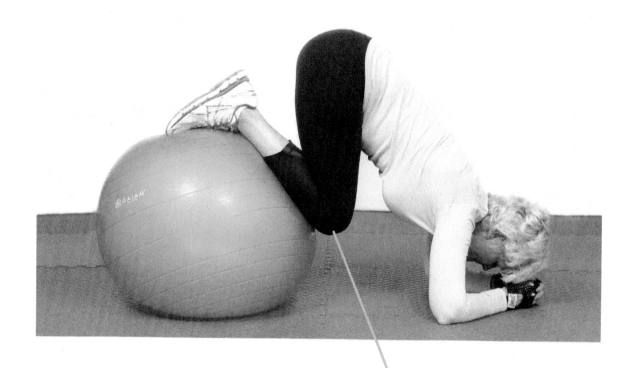

Leg position

Bring your knees toward
your chest as far as
possible.

Concluding Remarks

We hope this book has provided you with a thorough understanding of how to weight train without injury. Specifically, we hope you have learned the benefits (and dangers) of proper (and improper) weight training. Whether you're a novice, professional, or trainer, we're confident that the techniques we demonstrate will allow you to achieve a safer and more beneficial workout.

Thank you.

Fred Stellabotte
Rachel Straub, MS, CSCS
www.WeightTrainingWOI.com

JOURNAL AND REFERENCE ABBREVIATIONS

Am J Phys Med Rehabil	American Journal of Physical Medicine & Rehabilitation
Am J Sports Med	American Journal of Sports Medicine
Arch Phys Med Rehabil	Archives of Physical Medicine and Rehabilitation
Br J Sports Med	British Journal of Sports Medicine
Bull NYU Hosp Jt Dis	Bulletin of the NYU Hospital for Joint Diseases
Clin Orthop Relat Res	Clinical Orthopaedics and Related Research
Clin Sports Med	Clinics in Sports Medicine
Curr Sports Med Rep	Current Sports Medicine Reports
Dyn Med	Dynamic Medicine
Exerc Sport Sci Rev	Exercise and Sport Sciences Reviews
Isokinet Exerc Sci	Isokinetics and Exercise Science
JAMA	Journal of the American Medical Association
J Appl Biomech	Journal of Applied Biomechanics
J Appl Res Clin Exp Ther	Journal of Applied Research in Clinical and Experimental Therapeutics
J Athl Train	Journal of Athletic Training
J Aust Strength Cond	Journal of Australian Strength and Conditioning

J Electromyogr Kinesiol	Journal of Electromyography and Kinesiology
J Foot Ankle Res	Journal of Foot and Ankle Research
J Hand Ther	Journal of Hand Therapy
J Manipulative Physiol Ther	Journal of Manipulative and Physiological Therapeutics
J Orthop Res	Journal of Orthopaedic Research
J Orthop Sports Phys Ther	Journal of Orthopaedic and Sports Physical Therapy
J Shoulder Elbow Surg	Journal of Shoulder and Elbow Surgery
J Spinal Disord	Journal of Spinal Disorders & Techniques
J Sports Sci	Journal of Sports Sciences
J Strength Cond Res	Journal of Strength and Conditioning Research
Med Eng Phys	Medical Engineering & Physics
Med Sci Sports Exerc	Medicine & Science in Sports & Exercise
N Am J Sports Phys Ther	North American Journal of Sports Physical Therapy
Physiother Theory Pract	Physiotherapy Theory and Practice
Phys Sportsmed	Physician and Sportsmedicine
Phys Ther	Physical Therapy
Phys Ther Sport	Physical Therapy in Sport
Res Q Exerc Sport	Research Quarterly for Exercise and Sport
Spine	Spine
Sports Med	Sports Medicine
Strength Cond J	Strength and Conditioning Journal

ENDNOTES

INTRODUCTION

1. Kerr ZY, Collins CL, Comstock RD. Epidemiology of weight training-related injuries presenting to United States emergency departments, 1990 to 2007. *Am J Sports Med.* 2010;38(4):765-771. http://ajs.sagepub.com/content/38/4/765.abstract

2. Garber CE, Blissmer B, Deschenes MR, et al. American College of Sports Medicine position stand. Quantity and quality of exercise for developing and maintaining cardiorespiratory, musculoskeletal, and neuromotor fitness in apparently healthy adults: guidance for prescribing exercise. *Med Sci Sports Exerc.* 2011;43(7):1334-1359. http:// journals.lww.com/acsm-msse/Fulltext/2011/07000/Quantity_and_Quality_of_Exercise_ for_Developing.26.aspx

CHAPTER I: MAKING YOUR WORKOUT EFFICIENT

1. Garber CE, Blissmer B, Deschenes MR, et al. American College of Sports Medicine position stand. Quantity and quality of exercise for developing and maintaining cardiorespiratory, musculoskeletal, and neuromotor fitness in apparently healthy adults: guidance for prescribing exercise. *Med Sci Sports Exerc.* 2011;43(7):1334-1359. http:// journals.lww.com/acsm-msse/Fulltext/2011/07000/Quantity_and_Quality_of_Exercise_ for_Developing.26.aspx

2. American College of Sports Medicine position stand. Progression models in resistance training for healthy adults. *Med Sci Sports Exerc.* 2009;41(3):687-708. http://journals.lww. com/acsm-msse/Fulltext/2009/03000/Progression_Models_in_Resistance_Training_ for.26.aspx

3. Alcaraz PE, Sanchez-Lorente J, Blazevich AJ. Physical performance and cardiovascular responses to an acute bout of heavy resistance circuit training versus traditional strength training. *J Strength Cond Res.* 2008;22(3):667-671. http://journals.lww.com/nsca-jscr/ Abstract/2008/05000/Physical_Performance_and_Cardiovascular_Responses.3.aspx

253

4.   McGill SM. Low back exercises: evidence for improving exercise regimens. *Phys Ther*. 1998;78(7):754-765. http://ptjournal.apta.org/content/78/7/754.long

5.   Lewis PB, Ruby D, Bush-Joseph CA. Muscle soreness and delayed-onset muscle soreness. *Clin Sports Med*. 2012;31(2):255-262. http://www.sportsmed.theclinics.com/article/S0278-5919%2811%2900099-8/pdf

6.   Cheung K, Hume P, Maxwell L. Delayed onset muscle soreness : treatment strategies and performance factors. *Sports Med*. 2003;33(2):145-164. http://link.springer.com/article/10.2165%2F00007256-200333020-00005

CHAPTER 3: THE SQUAT

1.   Schoenfeld BJ. Squatting kinematics and kinetics and their application to exercise performance. *J Strength Cond Res*. 2010;24(12):3497-3506. http://journals.lww.com/nsca-jscr/Abstract/2010/12000/Squatting_Kinematics_and_Kinetics_and_Their.40.aspx

2.   Nagura T, Matsumoto H, Kiriyama Y, Chaudhari A, Andriacchi TP. Tibiofemoral joint contact force in deep knee flexion and its consideration in knee osteoarthritis and joint replacement. *J Appl Biomech*. 2006;22(4):305-313. http://www.ncbi.nlm.nih.gov/pubmed/17293627

3.   Escamilla RF. Knee biomechanics of the dynamic squat exercise. *Med Sci Sports Exerc*. 2001;33(1):127-141. http://journals.lww.com/acsm-msse/pages/articleviewer.aspx?year=2001&issue=01000&article=00020&type=abstract

4.   Russell PJ, Phillips SJ. A preliminary comparison of front and back squat exercises. *Res Q Exerc Sport*. 1989;60(3):201-208. http://www.tandfonline.com/doi/abs/10.1080/02701367.1989.10607441#.UrE0RfYwJ_Y

5.   Donnelly DV, Berg WP, Fiske DM. The effect of the direction of gaze on the kinematics of the squat exercise. *J Strength Cond Res*. 2006;20(1):145-150. http://journals.lww.com/nsca-jscr/Abstract/2006/02000/The_Effect_of_the_Direction_of_Gaze_on_the.23.aspx

6.   Caterisano A, Moss RF, Pellinger TK, et al. The effect of back squat depth on the EMG activity of 4 superficial hip and thigh muscles. *J Strength Cond Res*. 2002;16(3):428-432. http://journals.lww.com/nsca-jscr/Abstract/2002/08000/The_Effect_of_Back_Squat_Depth_on_the_EMG_Activity.14.aspx

7.   Wallace DA, Salem GJ, Salinas R, Powers CM. Patellofemoral joint kinetics while squatting with and without an external load. *J Orthop Sports Phys Ther*. 2002;32(4):141-148. http://www.jospt.org/doi/pdf/10.2519/jospt.2002.32.4.141

8.   Powers CM, Ho KY, Chen YJ, Souza RB, Farrokhi S. Patellofemoral joint stress during weight bearing and non-weight bearing quadriceps exercises. *J Orthop Sports Phys Ther*. 2014;44(5):320-327. http://www.jospt.org/doi/abs/10.2519/jospt.2014.4936?url_ver=Z39.882003&rfr_id=ori:rid:crossref.org&rfr_dat=cr_pub%3dpubmed&#.U0Mqk8cyluQ

9. Thambyah A, Goh JC, De SD. Contact stresses in the knee joint in deep flexion. *Med Eng Phys.* 2005;27(4):329-335. http://www.medengphys.com/article/S1350-4533%2804%2900167-5/abstract

10. Colado JC, García-Massó X. Technique and safety aspects of resistance exercises: a systematic review of the literature. *Phys Sportsmed.* 2009;37(2):104-111. http://www.tandfonline.com/doi/abs/10.3810/psm.2009.06.1716#.Veo4sXvTDWU

11. Escamilla RF, Zheng N, Macleod TD, et al. Patellofemoral joint force and stress during the wall squat and one-leg squat. *Med Sci Sports Exerc.* 2009;41(4):879-888. http://journals.lww.com/acsm-msse/Abstract/2009/04000/Patellofemoral_Joint_Force_and_Stress_during_the.18.aspx

12. Escamilla RF, Macleod TD, Wilk KE, Paulos L, Andrews JR. Anterior cruciate ligament strain and tensile forces for weight-bearing and non-weight-bearing exercises: a guide to exercise selection. *J Orthop Sports Phys Ther.* 2012;42(3):208-220. http://www.jospt.org/doi/pdf/10.2519/jospt.2012.3768

13. McKean MR, Burkett BJ. Knee behaviour in squatting. *J Aust Strength Cond.* 2012;20(2):23-36. http://www.strengthandconditioning.org/jasc-20-2-peer-review-knee-behaviour-in-squatting

14. Biscarini A, Benvenuti P, Botti F, Mastrandrea F, Zanuso S. Modelling the joint torques and loadings during squatting at the Smith machine. *J Sports Sci.* 2011;29(5):457-469. http://www.tandfonline.com/doi/abs/10.1080/02640414.2010.534859?url_ver=Z39.88-2003&rfr_id=ori:rid:crossref.org&rfr_dat=cr_pub%3dpubmed&#.UrEy5fYwJ_Y

15. Schwanbeck S, Chilibeck PD, Binsted G. A comparison of free weight squat to Smith machine squat using electromyography. *J Strength Cond Res.* 2009;23(9):2588-2591. http://journals.lww.com/nsca-jscr/Abstract/2009/12000/A_Comparison_of_Free_Weight_Squat_to_Smith_Machine.23.aspx

CHAPTER 4: THE LUNGE

1. Escamilla RF, Zheng N, Macleod TD, et al. Patellofemoral joint force and stress between a short- and long-step forward lunge. *J Orthop Sports Phys Ther.* 2008;38(11):681-690. http://www.jospt.org/doi/pdf/10.2519/jospt.2008.2694

2. Schoenfeld BJ. Squatting kinematics and kinetics and their application to exercise performance. *J Strength Cond Res.* 2010;24(12):3497-3506. http://journals.lww.com/nsca-jscr/Abstract/2010/12000/Squatting_Kinematics_and_Kinetics_and_Their.40.aspx

3. Escamilla RF, Zheng N, Macleod TD, et al. Patellofemoral joint force and stress during the wall squat and one-leg squat. *Med Sci Sports Exerc.* 2009;41(4):879-888. http://journals.lww.com/acsm-msse/Abstract/2009/04000/Patellofemoral_Joint_Force_and_Stress_during_the.18.aspx

4. Biscarini A, Benvenuti P, Botti F, Mastrandrea F, Zanuso S. Modelling the joint torques and loadings during squatting at the Smith machine. *J Sports Sci.* 2011;29(5):457-469. http://www.tandfonline.com/doi/abs/10.1080/02640414.2010.534859?url_ver=Z39.88-2003&rfr_id=ori:rid:crossref.org&rfr_dat=cr_pub%3dpubmed&#.UrEy5fYwJ_Y

5.   Escamilla RF, Macleod TD, Wilk KE, Paulos L, Andrews JR. Anterior cruciate ligament strain and tensile forces for weight-bearing and non-weight-bearing exercises: a guide to exercise selection. *J Orthop Sports Phys Ther*. 2012;42(3):208-220. http://www.jospt.org/doi/pdf/10.2519/jospt.2012.3768

6.   Farrokhi S, Pollard CD, Souza RB, Chen YJ, Reischl S, Powers CM. Trunk position influences the kinematics, kinetics, and muscle activity of the lead lower extremity during the forward lunge exercise. *J Orthop Sports Phys Ther*. 2008;38(7):403-409. http://www.jospt.org/doi/pdf/10.2519/jospt.2008.2634

7.   Calhoon G, Fry AC. Injury rates and profiles of elite competitive weightlifters. *J Athl Train*. 1999;34(3):232-238. http://www.ncbi.nlm.nih.gov/pmc/articles/PMC1322916/pdf/jathtrain00007-0016.pdf

CHAPTER 5: THE LEG PRESS

1.   Escamilla RF, Fleisig GS, Zheng N, et al. Effects of technique variations on knee biomechanics during the squat and leg press. *Med Sci Sports Exerc*. 2001;33(9):1552-1566. http://journals.lww.com/acsm-msse/Abstract/2001/09000/Effects_of_technique_variations_on_knee.20.aspx

2.   McGill S. *Low Back Disorders: Evidence Based Prevention and Rehabilitation*. 2nd ed. Champaign, Ill: Human Kinetics Publishers; 2007.

3.   Da Silva EM, Brentano MA, Cadore EL, De Almeida AP, Kruel LF. Analysis of muscle activation during different leg press exercises at submaximum effort levels. *J Strength Cond Res*. 2008;22(4):1059-1065. http://journals.lww.com/nsca-jscr/Abstract/2008/07000/Analysis_of_Muscle_Activation_During_Different_Leg.5.aspx

4.   Powers CM. The influence of abnormal hip mechanics on knee injury: a biomechanical perspective. *J Orthop Sports Phys Ther*. 2010;40(2):42-51. http://www.jospt.org/doi/pdf/10.2519/jospt.2010.3337

CHAPTER 6: THE LEG EXTENSION

1.   Glass R, Waddell J, Hoogenboom B. The effects of open versus closed kinetic chain exercises on patients with ACL deficient or reconstructed knees: a systematic review. *N Am J Sports Phys Ther*. 2010;5(2):74-84. http://www.ncbi.nlm.nih.gov/pmc/articles/PMC2953392/

2.   Witvrouw E, Danneels L, Van Tiggelen D, Willems TM, Cambier D. Open versus closed kinetic chain exercises in patellofemoral pain: a 5-year prospective randomized study. *Am J Sports Med*. 2004;32(5):1122-1130. http://ajs.sagepub.com/content/32/5/1122.abstract?sid=7d787a18-3014-49ef-9415-2aa9636c3737

3.   Cohen ZA, Roglic H, Grelsamer RP, et al. Patellofemoral stresses during open and closed kinetic chain exercises. An analysis using computer simulation. *Am J Sports Med.* 2001;29(4):480-487. http://ajs.sagepub.com/content/29/4/480.abstract?sid=550d5872-5c65-4069-9c6b-812a31f95fbe

4.   Powers CM, Ho KY, Chen YJ, Souza RB, Farrokhi S. Patellofemoral joint stress during weight bearing and non-weight bearing quadriceps exercises. *J Orthop Sports Phys Ther.* 2014;44(5):320-327. http://www.jospt.org/doi/abs/10.2519/jospt.2014.4936?url_ver=Z39.882003&rfr_id=ori:rid:crossref.org&rfr_dat=cr_pub%3dpubmed&#.U0Mqk8cyluQ

5.   Li G, Zayontz S, DeFrate LE, Most E, Suggs JF, Rubash HE. Kinematics of the knee at high flexion angles: an in vitro investigation. *J Orthop Res.* 2004;22(1):90-95. http://onlinelibrary.wiley.com/doi/10.1016/S0736-0266%2803%2900118-9/abstract;jsessionid=7DBC4DFA38A44946F22B9B0CB8918703.f01t03

6.   Thambyah A, Goh JC, De SD. Contact stresses in the knee joint in deep flexion. *Med Eng Phys.* 2005;27(4):329-335. http://www.medengphys.com/article/S1350-4533%2804%2900167-5/abstract

7.   Colado JC, García-Massó X. Technique and safety aspects of resistance exercises: a systematic review of the literature. *Phys Sportsmed.* 2009;37(2):104-111. http://www.tandfonline.com/doi/abs/10.3810/psm.2009.06.1716#.Veo4sXvTDWU

8.   Steinkamp LA, Dillingham MF, Markel MD, Hill JA, Kaufman KR. Biomechanical considerations in patellofemoral joint rehabilitation. *Am J Sports Med.* 1993;21(3):438-444. http://ajs.sagepub.com/content/21/3/438.abstract?sid=aaa9b68b-b953-45eb-ab71-0825bf389435

CHAPTER 7: THE LEG CURL

1.   Opar DA, Williams MD, Shield AJ. Hamstring strain injuries: factors that lead to injury and re-injury. *Sports Med.* 2012;42(3):209-226. http://link.springer.com/article/10.2165%2F11594800-000000000-00000

2.   Wright GA, Delong TH, Gehlsen G. Electromyographic activity of the hamstrings during performance of the leg curl, stiff-leg deadlift, and, back squat movements. *J Strength Cond Res.* 1999;13(2):168-174. http://journals.lww.com/nsca-jscr/Abstract/1999/05000/Electromyographic_Activity_of_the_Hamstrings.12.aspx

3.   Gardner P, Cole DE. The stiff-legged deadlift. *Strength Cond J.* 1999;21(5):7-14. http://journals.lww.com/nsca-scj/Citation/1999/10000/The_Stiff_Legged_Deadlift.1.aspx

4.   Garrett WE, Jr. Muscle strain injuries: clinical and basic aspects. *Med Sci Sports Exerc.* 1990;22(4):436-443. http://journals.lww.com/acsm-msse/Abstract/1990/08000/Muscle_strain_injuries__clinical_and_basic_aspects.3.aspx

5.   Kaminski TW, Wabbersen CV, Murphy RM. Concentric versus enhanced eccentric hamstring strength training: clinical implications. *J Athl Train.* 1998;33(3):216-221. http://www.ncbi.nlm.nih.gov/pmc/articles/PMC1320426/

CHAPTER 8: THE CALF RAISE

1.   Chang HJ, Burke AE, Glass RM. JAMA patient page. Achilles tendinopathy. *JAMA.* 2010;303(2):188. http://jama.jamanetwork.com/article.aspx?articleid=185201
2.   Sussmilch-Leitch SP, Collins NJ, Bialocerkowski AE, Warden SJ, Crossley KM. Physical therapies for Achilles tendinopathy: systematic review and meta-analysis. *J Foot Ankle Res.* 2012;5(1):15. http://www.jfootankleres.com/content/5/1/15
3.   Hebert-Losier K, Schneiders AG, Newsham-West RJ, Sullivan SJ. Scientific bases and clinical utilisation of the calf-raise test. *Phys Ther Sport.* 2009;10(4):142-149. http://www.ncbi.nlm.nih.gov/pubmed/?term=Scientific+bases+and+clinical+utilisation+of+the+calf-raise+test

CHAPTER 9: THE LAT PULLDOWN

1.   Lusk SJ, Hale BD, Russell DM. Grip width and forearm orientation effects on muscle activity during the lat pull-down. *J Strength Cond Res.* 2010;24(7):1895-1900. http://journals.lww.com/nsca-jscr/pages/articleviewer.aspx?year=2010&issue=07000&article=00027&type=abstract
2.   Signorile JF, Zink AJ, Szwed SP. A comparative electromyographical investigation of muscle utilization patterns using various hand positions during the lat pull-down. *J Strength Cond Res.* 2002;16(4):539-546. http://journals.lww.com/nsca-jscr/Abstract/2002/11000/A_Comparative_Electromyographical_Investigation_of.8.aspx
3.   Fees M, Decker T, Snyder-Mackler L, Axe MJ. Upper extremity weight-training modifications for the injured athlete. A clinical perspective. *Am J Sports Med.* 1998;26(5):732-742. http://ajs.sagepub.com/content/26/5/732.abstract?sid=411bb4d3-6bca-4ddd-ba3a-d36e55e2c0f2

CHAPTER 10: THE ROW

1.   Lehman GJ, Buchan DD, Lundy A, Myers N, Nalborczyk A. Variations in muscle activation levels during traditional latissimus dorsi weight training exercises: An experimental study. *Dyn Med.* 2004;3(1):4. http://www.ncbi.nlm.nih.gov/pmc/articles/PMC449729/
2.   Fenwick CM, Brown SH, McGill SM. Comparison of different rowing exercises: trunk muscle activation and lumbar spine motion, load, and stiffness. *J Strength Cond Res.* 2009;23(5):1408-1417. http://journals.lww.com/nsca-jscr/Abstract/2009/08000/Comparison_of_Different_Rowing_Exercises__Trunk.7.aspx
3.   Durall CJ, Manske RC, Davies GJ. Avoiding shoulder injury from resistance training. *Strength Cond J.* 2001;23(5):10-18. http://journals.lww.com/nsca-scj/Citation/2001/10000/Avoiding_Shoulder_Injury_From_Resistance_Training.2.aspx

CHAPTER 11: THE REVERSE FLY

1. Escamilla RF, Yamashiro K, Paulos L, Andrews JR. Shoulder muscle activity and function in common shoulder rehabilitation exercises. *Sports Med.* 2009;39(8):663-685. http://link.springer.com/article/10.2165%2F00007256-200939080-00004

2. Durall CJ, Manske RC, Davies GJ. Avoiding shoulder injury from resistance training. *Strength Cond J.* 2001;23(5):10-18. http://journals.lww.com/nsca-scj/Citation/2001/10000/Avoiding_Shoulder_Injury_From_Resistance_Training.2.aspx

CHAPTER 12: THE LOW-BACK EXTENSION

1. Kendall FP, McCreary EK, Provance PG, Rodgers MM, Romani WA. *Muscles: Testing and Function with Posture and Pain.* 5th ed. Baltimore, MD: Lippincott Williams & Wilkins; 2005.

2. McGill S. *Low Back Disorders: Evidence Based Prevention and Rehabilitation.* 2nd ed. Champaign, Ill: Human Kinetics Publishers; 2007.

3. McGill SM. Low back exercises: evidence for improving exercise regimens. *Phys Ther.* 1998;78(7):754-765. http://ptjournal.apta.org/content/78/7/754.long

4. Walker BF. The prevalence of low back pain: a systematic review of the literature from 1966 to 1998. *J Spinal Disord.* 2000;13(3):205-217. http://journals.lww.com/jspinaldisorders/Abstract/2000/06000/The_Prevalence_of_Low_Back_Pain__A_Systematic.3.aspx

5. Reiman MP, Bolgla LA, Loudon JK. A literature review of studies evaluating gluteus maximus and gluteus medius activation during rehabilitation exercises. *Physiother Theory Pract.* 2012;28(4):257-268. http://informahealthcare.com/doi/abs/10.3109/09593985.2011.604981

6. Calhoon G, Fry AC. Injury rates and profiles of elite competitive weightlifters. *J Athl Train.* 1999;34(3):232-238. http://www.ncbi.nlm.nih.gov/pmc/articles/PMC1322916/pdf/jathtrain00007-0016.pdf

7. Powers CM, Beneck GJ, Kulig K, Landel RF, Fredericson M. Effects of a single session of posterior-to-anterior spinal mobilization and press-up exercise on pain response and lumbar spine extension in people with nonspecific low back pain. *Phys Ther.* 2008;88(4):485-493. http://ptjournal.apta.org/content/88/4/485.long

8. Larsen K, Weidick F, Leboeuf-Yde C. Can passive prone extensions of the back prevent back problems? A randomized, controlled intervention trial of 314 military conscripts. *Spine.* 2002;27(24):2747-2752. http://journals.lww.com/spinejournal/pages/articleviewer.aspx?year=2002&issue=12150&article=00002&type=abstract

CHAPTER 13: THE BENCH PRESS

1.   Kuzmits FE, Adams AJ. The NFL combine: does it predict performance in the National Football League? *J Strength Cond Res.* 2008;22(6):1721-1727. http://journals.lww.com/nsca-jscr/Abstract/2008/11000/The_NFL_Combine__Does_It_Predict_Performance_in.1.aspx

2.   Santana JC, Vera-Garcia FJ, McGill SM. A kinetic and electromyographic comparison of the standing cable press and bench press. *J Strength Cond Res.* 2007;21(4):1271-1277. http://journals.lww.com/nsca-jscr/Abstract/2007/11000/A_Kinetic_and_Electromyographic_Comparison_of_the.50.aspx

3.   Raske A, Norlin R. Injury incidence and prevalence among elite weight and power lifters. *Am J Sports Med.* 2002;30(2):248-256. http://ajs.sagepub.com/content/30/2/248.abstract?sid=11e22a4a-6e7f-4242-84b2-395185459ef7

4.   Kolber MJ, Beekhuizen KS, Cheng MS, Hellman MA. Shoulder injuries attributed to resistance training: a brief review. *J Strength Cond Res.* 2010;24(6):1696-1704. http://journals.lww.com/nsca-jscr/Abstract/2010/06000/Shoulder_Injuries_Attributed_to_Resistance.36.aspx

5.   Durall CJ, Manske RC, Davies GJ. Avoiding shoulder injury from resistance training. *Strength Cond J.* 2001;23(5):10-18. http://journals.lww.com/nsca-scj/Citation/2001/10000/Avoiding_Shoulder_Injury_From_Resistance_Training.2.aspx

6.   Bhatia DN, de Beer JF, van Rooyen KS, Lam F, du Toit DF. The "bench-presser's shoulder": an overuse insertional tendinopathy of the pectoralis minor muscle. *Br J Sports Med.* 2007;41(8):e1-e4. http://www.ncbi.nlm.nih.gov/pmc/articles/PMC2465431/

7.   Fees M, Decker T, Snyder-Mackler L, Axe MJ. Upper extremity weight-training modifications for the injured athlete. A clinical perspective. *Am J Sports Med.* 1998;26(5):732-742. http://ajs.sagepub.com/content/26/5/732.abstract?sid=3955e78e-9521-4d7a-9885-f677dde98fff

8.   Green CM, Comfort P. The affect of grip width on bench press performance and risk of injury. *Strength Cond J.* 2007;29(5):10-14. http://journals.lww.com/nsca-scj/Abstract/2007/10000/The_Affect_of_Grip_Width_on_Bench_Press.1.aspx

9.   Lehman GJ. The influence of grip width and forearm pronation/supination on upper-body myoelectric activity during the flat bench press. *J Strength Cond Res.* 2005;19(3):587-591. http://journals.lww.com/nsca-jscr/Abstract/2005/08000/The_Influence_of_Grip_Width_and_Forearm.17.aspx

10.   Trebs AA, Brandenburg JP, Pitney WA. An electromyography analysis of 3 muscles surrounding the shoulder joint during the performance of a chest press exercise at several angles. *J Strength Cond Res.* 2010;24(7):1925-1930. http://journals.lww.com/nsca-jscr/Abstract/2010/07000/An_Electromyography_Analysis_of_3_Muscles.31.aspx

11.   Schick EE, Coburn JW, Brown LE, et al. A comparison of muscle activation between a Smith machine and free weight bench press. *J Strength Cond Res.* 2010;24(3):779-784. http://journals.lww.com/nsca-jscr/Abstract/2010/03000/A_Comparison_of_Muscle_Activation_Between_a_Smith.26.aspx

CHAPTER 14: THE CHEST FLY

1. Kolber MJ, Beekhuizen KS, Cheng MS, Hellman MA. Shoulder injuries attributed to resistance training: a brief review. *J Strength Cond Res.* 2010;24(6):1696-1704. http://journals.lww.com/nsca-jscr/Abstract/2010/06000/Shoulder_Injuries_Attributed_to_Resistance.36.aspx

2. Durall CJ, Manske RC, Davies GJ. Avoiding shoulder injury from resistance training. *Strength Cond J.* 2001;23(5):10-18. http://journals.lww.com/nsca-scj/Citation/2001/10000/Avoiding_Shoulder_Injury_From_Resistance_Training.2.aspx

CHAPTER 15: THE SHOULDER PRESS

1. Kolber MJ, Beekhuizen KS, Cheng MS, Hellman MA. Shoulder injuries attributed to resistance training: a brief review. *J Strength Cond Res.* 2010;24(6):1696-1704. http://journals.lww.com/nsca-jscr/Abstract/2010/06000/Shoulder_Injuries_Attributed_to_Resistance.36.aspx

2. Calhoon G, Fry AC. Injury rates and profiles of elite competitive weightlifters. *J Athl Train.* 1999;34(3):232-238. http://www.ncbi.nlm.nih.gov/pmc/articles/PMC1322916/pdf/jathtrain00007-0016.pdf

3. Barlow JC, Benjamin BW, Birt P, Hughes CJ. Shoulder strength and range-of-motion characteristics in bodybuilders. *J Strength Cond Res.* 2002;16(3):367-372. http://journals.lww.com/nsca-jscr/Abstract/2002/08000/Shoulder_Strength_and_Range_Of_Motion.6.aspx

4. Paoli A, Marcolin G, Petrone N. Influence of different ranges of motion on selective recruitment of shoulder muscles in the sitting military press: an electromyographic study. *J Strength Cond Res.* 2010;24(6):1578-1583. http://journals.lww.com/nsca-jscr/pages/articleviewer.aspx?year=2010&issue=06000&article=00021&type=abstract

5. Fees M, Decker T, Snyder-Mackler L, Axe MJ. Upper extremity weight-training modifications for the injured athlete. A clinical perspective. *Am J Sports Med.* 1998;26(5):732-742. http://ajs.sagepub.com/content/26/5/732.abstract?sid=3955e78e-9521-4d7a-9885-f677dde98fff

6. Durall CJ, Manske RC, Davies GJ. Avoiding shoulder injury from resistance training. *Strength Cond J.* 2001;23(5):10-18. http://journals.lww.com/nsca-scj/Citation/2001/10000/Avoiding_Shoulder_Injury_From_Resistance_Training.2.aspx

CHAPTER 16: THE SHOULDER RAISE

1. Paoli A, Marcolin G, Petrone N. Influence of different ranges of motion on selective recruitment of shoulder muscles in the sitting military press: an electromyographic study. *J Strength Cond Res.* 2010;24(6):1578-1583. http://journals.lww.com/nsca-jscr/pages/articleviewer.aspx?year=2010&issue=06000&article=00021&type=abstract

2. Kolber MJ, Beekhuizen KS, Cheng MS, Hellman MA. Shoulder injuries attributed to resistance training: a brief review. *J Strength Cond Res.* 2010;24(6):1696-1704. http://journals.lww.com/nsca-jscr/Abstract/2010/06000/Shoulder_Injuries_Attributed_to_Resistance.36.aspx

3. Burke WS, Vangsness CT, Powers CM. Strengthening the supraspinatus: a clinical and biomechanical review. *Clin Orthop Relat Res.* 2002(402):292-298. http://journals.lww.com/corr/Abstract/2002/09000/Strengthening_the_Supraspinatus__A_Clinical_and.30.aspx

4. Culham E, Peat M. Functional anatomy of the shoulder complex. *J Orthop Sports Phys Ther.* 1993;18(1):342-342. http://www.jospt.org/doi/pdf/10.2519/jospt.1993.18.1.342

5. Hellwig EV, Perrin D. A comparison of two positions for assessing shoulder rotator peak torque: the traditional frontal plane versus the plane of the scapula. *Isokinet Exerc Sci.* 1991;1(4):202-206. http://iospress.metapress.com/content/5555127877qkvm44/?p=3b97f619dc9b4edeb769808239fcc5ad&pi=0

6. Durall CJ, Manske RC, Davies GJ. Avoiding shoulder injury from resistance training. *Strength Cond J.* 2001;23(5):10-18. http://journals.lww.com/nsca-scj/Citation/2001/10000/Avoiding_Shoulder_Injury_From_Resistance_Training.2.aspx

7. Escamilla RF, Yamashiro K, Paulos L, Andrews JR. Shoulder muscle activity and function in common shoulder rehabilitation exercises. *Sports Med.* 2009;39(8):663-685. http://link.springer.com/article/10.2165%2F00007256-200939080-00004

CHAPTER 17: THE BICEPS CURL

1. Raske A, Norlin R. Injury incidence and prevalence among elite weight and power lifters. *Am J Sports Med.* 2002;30(2):248-256. http://ajs.sagepub.com/content/30/2/248.abstract?sid=9783874b-d438-4613-b318-3956f742c5e3

2. Ciccotti MG, Charlton WP. Epicondylitis in the athlete. *Clin Sports Med.* 2001;20(1):77-93. http://www.sciencedirect.com/science/article/pii/S0278591905702489

3. Rokito AS, Iofin I. Simultaneous bilateral distal biceps tendon rupture during a Preacher Curl exercise: a case report. *Bull NYU Hosp Jt Dis.* 2008;66(1):68-71. http://www.nwoa.com/wordpress/wp-content/uploads/2011/12/Bilateral-Distal-Biceps.pdf

4. Badia A, Stennett C. Sports-related injuries of the elbow. *J Hand Ther.* 2006;19(2):206-226. http://www.sciencedirect.com/science/article/pii/S0894113006000470

5. Rettig AC. Elbow, forearm and wrist injuries in the athlete. *Sports Med.* 1998;25(2):115-130. http://link.springer.com/article/10.2165%2F00007256-199825020-00004

6.   de Serres SJ, Hebert LJ, Arsenault AB, Goulet C. Effect of pronation and supination tasks on elbow flexor muscles. *J Electromyogr Kinesiol.* 1992;2(1):53-58. http://www.sciencedirect.com/science/article/pii/1050641192900087

7.   Bechtel R, Caldwell GE. The influence of task and angle on torque production and muscle activity at the elbow. *J Electromyogr Kinesiol.* 1994;4(4):195-204. http://www.sciencedirect.com/science/article/pii/1050641194900078

8.   Dupont L, Gamet D, Perot C. Motor unit recruitment and EMG power spectra during ramp contractions of a bifunctional muscle. *J Electromyogr Kinesiol.* 2000;10(4):217-224. http://www.sciencedirect.com/science/article/pii/S1050641100000146

CHAPTER 19: THE CRUNCH

1.   Akuthota V, Ferreiro A, Moore T, Fredericson M. Core stability exercise principles. *Curr Sports Med Rep.* 2008;7(1):39-44. http://journals.lww.com/acsm-csmr/pages/articleviewer.aspx?year=2008&issue=01000&article=00014&type=abstract

2.   Hamlyn N, Behm DG, Young WB. Trunk muscle activation during dynamic weight-training exercises and isometric instability activities. *J Strength Cond Res.* 2007;21(4):1108-1112. http://journals.lww.com/nsca-jscr/Abstract/2007/11000/Trunk_Muscle_Activation_During_Dynamic.22.aspx

3.   Monfort-Panego M, Vera-Garcia FJ, Sanchez-Zuriaga D, Sarti-Martinez MA. Electromyographic studies in abdominal exercises: a literature synthesis. *J Manipulative Physiol Ther.* 2009;32(3):232-244. http://www.jmptonline.org/article/S0161-4754%2809%2900053-0/abstract

4.   Escamilla RF, Babb E, DeWitt R, et al. Electromyographic analysis of traditional and nontraditional abdominal exercises: implications for rehabilitation and training. *Phys Ther.* 2006;86(5):656-671. http://ptjournal.apta.org/content/86/5/656.long

5.   McGill SM. Low back exercises: evidence for improving exercise regimens. *Phys Ther.* 1998;78(7):754-765. http://ptjournal.apta.org/content/78/7/754.long

6.   Anders M. New study puts the crunch on ineffective ab exercises. *ACE Fitness Matters.* 2001;7(3):9-11. https://www.acefitness.org/getfit/studies/bestworstabexercises.pdf

7.   Petrofsky JS, Batt J, Davis N, et al. Core muscle activity during exercise on a mini stability ball compared with abdominal crunches on the floor and on a swiss ball. *J Appl Res Clin Exp Ther.* 2007;7(3):255. http://jrnlappliedresearch.com/articles/Vol7Iss3/PetrofskyVol7No3.pdf

CHAPTER 20: THE LEG RAISE

1.   Escamilla RF, Babb E, DeWitt R, et al. Electromyographic analysis of traditional and nontraditional abdominal exercises: implications for rehabilitation and training. *Phys Ther.* 2006;86(5):656-671. http://ptjournal.apta.org/content/86/5/656.long

2.   Barr KP, Griggs M, Cadby T. Lumbar stabilization: core concepts and current literature, Part 1. *Am J Phys Med Rehabil.* 2005;84(6):473-480. http://journals.lww.com/ajpmr/pages/articleviewer.aspx?year=2005&issue=06000&article=00012&type=abstract

3.   Krause DA, Youdas JW, Hollman JH, Smith J. Abdominal muscle performance as measured by the double leg-lowering test. *Arch Phys Med Rehabil.* 2005;86(7):1345-1348. http://www.archives-pmr.org/article/S0003-9993%2805%2900086-9/fulltext

4.   Axler CT, McGill SM. Low back loads over a variety of abdominal exercises: searching for the safest abdominal challenge. *Med Sci Sports Exerc.* 1997;29(6):804-811. http://journals.lww.com/acsm-msse/Abstract/1997/06000/Low_back_loads_over_a_variety_of_abdominal.11.aspx

CHAPTER 21: THE PLANK

1.   Schellenberg KL, Lang JM, Chan KM, Burnham RS. A clinical tool for office assessment of lumbar spine stabilization endurance: prone and supine bridge maneuvers. *Am J Phys Med Rehabil.* 2007;86(5):380-386. http://journals.lww.com/ajpmr/pages/articleviewer.aspx?year=2007&issue=05000&article=00009&type=abstract

2.   McGill SM. Low back stability: from formal description to issues for performance and rehabilitation. *Exerc Sport Sci Rev.* 2001;29(1):26-31. http://journals.lww.com/acsm-essr/pages/articleviewer.aspx?year=2001&issue=01000&article=00006&type=abstract

3.   Youdas JW, Budach BD, Ellerbusch JV, Stucky CM, Wait KR, Hollman JH. Comparison of muscle-activation patterns during the conventional push-up and perfect pushup exercises. *J Strength Cond Res.* 2010;24(12):3352-3362. http://journals.lww.com/nsca-jscr/Abstract/2010/12000/Comparison_of_Muscle_Activation_Patterns_During.21.aspx

4.   Freeman S, Karpowicz A, Gray J, McGill S. Quantifying muscle patterns and spine load during various forms of the push-up. *Med Sci Sports Exerc.* 2006;38(3):570-577. http://journals.lww.com/acsm-msse/Abstract/2006/03000/Quantifying_Muscle_Patterns_and_Spine_Load_during.24.aspx

5.   Escamilla RF, Lewis C, Bell D, et al. Core muscle activation during swiss ball and traditional abdominal exercises. *J Orthop Sports Phys Ther.* 2010;40(5):265-276. http://www.jospt.org/doi/pdf/10.2519/jospt.2010.3073

6.   McGill S. Core training: Evidence translating to better performance and injury prevention. *Strength Cond J.* 2010;32(3):33-46. http://journals.lww.com/nsca-scj/Abstract/2010/06000/Core_Training__Evidence_Translating_to_Better.4.aspx

ABOUT THE AUTHORS

Fred Stellabotte, a US Navy vetern and an expert in bodybuilding, has developed weight-training programs with a focus on proper form and injury prevention for over 50 years. He has trained movie stars, champion bodybuilders, professional athletes (including Los Angeles Dodgers baseball team and Oakland Raiders football team players), and members of the general public. From 1970 to 1989, he founded and directed southern California's Manhattan Beach Athletic Club for Men and the Manhattan Beach Athletic Club for Women, two of the largest facilities of their kind in America. His

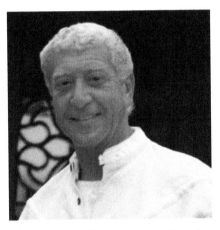

knowledge and experience result from years of research, including study with monks who practice martial arts in China; extensive coursework in kinesiology, anatomy, and neurology; and scrutiny of proper muscle function through examination of his own body in front of mirrors. *Weight Training Without Injury*, co-authored by one of his star students, Rachel Straub, is Fred's legacy. It shares his knowledge, acquired over a lifetime, with future generations.

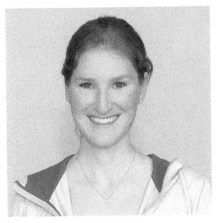

Rachel Straub, MS, CSCS, is a Phi Beta Kappa graduate of Carnegie Mellon, where she received her BA in chemistry with university and research honors. She holds master's degrees in exercise physiology and nutritional sciences from San Diego State University and a third master's degree in biokinesiology (with a focus on biomechanics) from the University of Southern California. She has been certified as a strength and conditioning specialist by the National Strength and Conditioning Association and is the co-author of scientific papers in the fields of biomechanics, sports medicine, nutrition, and computational chemistry, published in the American Journal of Sports Medicine, Journal of Strength and Conditioning Research, Journal of Electromyography and

Kinesiology, Nutrition Research, and Physical Biology and other journals. Rachel, a skilled investor, currently co-manages extensive brokerage accounts that are outperforming benchmark indices such as the S&P 500 and NASDAQ Composite.

Visit the authors at www.WeightTrainingWOI.com
or contact them by sending an email to info@weighttrainingwoi.com.

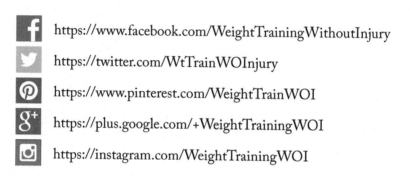

https://www.facebook.com/WeightTrainingWithoutInjury

https://twitter.com/WtTrainWOInjury

https://www.pinterest.com/WeightTrainWOI

https://plus.google.com/+WeightTrainingWOI

https://instagram.com/WeightTrainingWOI

INDEX

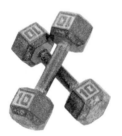

CPSIA information can be obtained
at www.ICGtesting.com
Printed in the USA
BVOW10s1948011116

466643BV00006B/16/P

9 780996 263818